T0258978

Oncology and COVID-19

Those affected by cancer or receiving cancer treatment have often been more susceptible to infections due to coexisting chronic diseases, overall poor health status, and systemic immunosuppressive states caused by both cancer and anticancer treatments. This pioneering text is an introduction to the key topics in the relationship between infection, pollution, and cancer and is an invaluable resource for residents and junior faculty in Oncology facing the practical problems arising and for those still in training.

- Looks at the lessons to be learned for future Oncology patients from a series of studies
- Presents relevant international experience from Oncology clinicians and researchers
- Brings together input from different countries, systems, and specialties

Oncology and COVID-19

Impact of the Pandemic on Patients and Treatments

Edited by
Luigi Cavanna
Chiara Citterio
Gabriella Marfe
Luigi Montano

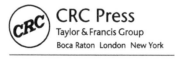

CRC Press
Taylor & Francis Group
Boca Raton London New York

CRC Press is an imprint of the
Taylor & Francis Group, an **informa** business

Designed cover image: Shutterstock

First edition published 2024
by CRC Press
6000 Broken Sound Parkway NW, Suite 300, Boca Raton, FL 33487-2742

and by CRC Press
4 Park Square, Milton Park, Abingdon, Oxon, OX14 4RN

CRC Press is an imprint of Taylor & Francis Group, LLC

© 2024 selection and editorial matter, Luigi Cavanna, Chiara Citterio, Gabriella Marfe, and Luigi Montano; individual chapters, the contributors

This book contains information obtained from authentic and highly regarded sources. While all reasonable efforts have been made to publish reliable data and information, neither the author[s] nor the publisher can accept any legal responsibility or liability for any errors or omissions that may be made. The publishers wish to make clear that any views or opinions expressed in this book by individual editors, authors or contributors are personal to them and do not necessarily reflect the views/opinions of the publishers. The information or guidance contained in this book is intended for use by medical, scientific or health-care professionals and is provided strictly as a supplement to the medical or other professional's own judgement, their knowledge of the patient's medical history, relevant manufacturer's instructions and the appropriate best practice guidelines. Because of the rapid advances in medical science, any information or advice on dosages, procedures or diagnoses should be independently verified. The reader is strongly urged to consult the relevant national drug formulary and the drug companies' and device or material manufacturers' printed instructions, and their websites, before administering or utilizing any of the drugs, devices or materials mentioned in this book. This book does not indicate whether a particular treatment is appropriate or suitable for a particular individual. Ultimately it is the sole responsibility of the medical professional to make his or her own professional judgements, so as to advise and treat patients appropriately. The authors and publishers have also attempted to trace the copyright holders of all material reproduced in this publication and apologize to copyright holders if permission to publish in this form has not been obtained. If any copyright material has not been acknowledged please write and let us know so we may rectify in any future reprint.

Except as permitted under U.S. Copyright Law, no part of this book may be reprinted, reproduced, transmitted, or utilized in any form by any electronic, mechanical, or other means, now known or hereafter invented, including photocopying, microfilming, and recording, or in any information storage or retrieval system, without written permission from the publishers.

For permission to photocopy or use material electronically from this work, access www.copyright.com or contact the Copyright Clearance Center, Inc. (CCC), 222 Rosewood Drive, Danvers, MA 01923, 978-750-8400. For works that are not available on CCC please contact mpkbookspermissions@tandf.co.uk

Trademark notice: Product or corporate names may be trademarks or registered trademarks and are used only for identification and explanation without intent to infringe.

ISBN: 978-1-032-42384-5 (hbk)
ISBN: 978-1-032-42383-8 (pbk)
ISBN: 978-1-003-36256-2 (ebk)

DOI: 10.1201/9781003362562

Typeset in Times
by SPi Technologies India Pvt Ltd (Straive)

Contents

Editors

Luigi Cavanna
Chief of Internal Medicine and
    Oncology
Casa di Cura Piacenza
Piacenza, Italy

Chiara Citterio
Oncology & Haematology Department,
    Oncology Unit
Piacenza General Hospital
Piacenza, Italy

Gabriella Marfe
Department of Scienze
    e Tecnologie Ambientali,
    Biologiche e Farmaceutiche
University of Campania
    "Luigi Vanvitelli"
Caserta, Italy

Luigi Montano
Head, Andrology Unit and Service of
    LifeStyle Medicine in UroAndrology
Local Health Authority (ASL) Salerno
Coordination Unit of the Network for
    Environmental and Reproductive
    Health (EcoFoodFertility Project),
    "S. Francis Hospital"
Oliveto Citra, Italy

Contributors

Mohammed Tanvir Ahammed
Department of Pediatric Hematology
 and Oncology
Dhaka Medical College Hospital
Dhaka, Bangladesh

Mehnaz Akter
Department of Pediatric Hematology
 and Oncology
Dhaka Medical College Hospital
Dhaka, Bangladesh

Massimo Ambroggi
Oncology Unit, Oncology and
 Hematology Department
Piacenza General Hospital
Piacenza, Italy

Elisa Anselmi
Oncology Unit, Oncology and
 Hematology Department
Piacenza General Hospital
Piacenza, Italy

Zannat Ara
Department of Pediatric Hematology
 and Oncology
Dhaka Medical College Hospital
Dhaka, Bangladesh

Nicoletta Bacchetta
Oncology Unit, Oncology and
 Hematology Department
Piacenza General Hospital
Piacenza, Italy

AKM Khairul Basher
Department of Pediatric Surgery
Dhaka Medical College Hospital
Dhaka, Bangladesh

Sachidanand Jee Bharati
Department of Onco-anaesthesia and
 Palliative Medicine
Dr Br Ambedkar Institute Rotary Cancer
 Hospital, All India Institute of
 Medical Sciences
Delhi, India

Claudia Biasini
Oncology Unit, Oncology and
 Hematology Department
Piacenza General Hospital
Piacenza, Italy

Nika Bric
Epidemiology and Cancer Registry
Institute of Oncology Ljubljana
Ljubljana, Slovenia

Carlo Brogna
Carlo Brogna, Craniomed Group srl
Montemiletto, Italy

Abhijit Chakraborty
Baylor College of Medicine and Texas
 Heart Institute
Houston, Texas, USA

Maria Luisia Chiusano
Department of Agriculture
University Federico II of Naples
Napoli, Italy

Gabriele Cremona
Oncology Unit, Oncology and
 Hematology Department
Piacenza General Hospital
Piacenza, Italy

Giulia Claire Giudice
Oncology Unit, Oncology and
    Hematology Department
Piacenza General Hospital
Piacenza, Italy

Marie Grill
Departments of Neurology,
Mayo Clinic and Mayo Clinic
    Cancer Center
Phoenix, Arizona, USA

Ehab Harahsheh
Departments of Neurology,
Mayo Clinic and Mayo Clinic
    Cancer Center
Phoenix, Arizona, USA

Nicola Inzerilli
Oncology Unit, Oncology and
    Hematology Department,
Piacenza General Hospital
Piacenza, Italy

Shahnoor Islam
Department of Pediatric Surgery
Dhaka Medical College Hospital
Dhaka, Bangladesh

Katarina Lokar
Epidemiology and Cancer Registry
Institute of Oncology Ljubljana
Ljubljana, Slovenia

Kenneth Lundstrom
PanTherapeutics
Lutry, Switzerland

Ana Mihor
Epidemiology and Cancer Registry
Institute of Oncology Ljubljana
Ljubljana, Slovenia

Giovanna Mirone
Department of Scienze e Tecnologie
    Ambientali
Biologiche e Farmaceutiche, University
    of Campania "Luigi Vanvitelli"
Caserta, Italy

AKM Amirul Morshed
Department of Pediatric Hematology
    and Oncology
Dhaka Medical College Hospital
Dhaka, Bangladesh

Maciej M Mrugala
Departments of Neurology and
    Oncology
Mayo Clinic and Mayo Clinic
    Cancer Center
Phoenix, Arizona, USA

Monica Muroni
Oncology Unit, Oncology and
    Hematology Department
Piacenza General Hospital
Piacenza, Italy

Kamrun Nahar
Department of Pediatric Surgery
Dhaka Medical College Hospital
Dhaka, Bangladesh

Camilla Di Nunzio
Oncology Unit, Oncology and
    Hematology Department
Piacenza General Hospital
Piacenza, Italy

Elena Orlandi
Oncology Unit, Oncology and
    Hematology Department
Piacenza General Hospital
Piacenza, Italy

Stefania Perna
Department of Scienze e Tecnologie
    Ambientali
Biologiche e Farmaceutiche, University
    of Campania "Luigi Vanvitelli"
Caserta, Italy

Marina Piscopo
Department of Biology
University Federico II of Naples
Napoli, Italy

Chandra Prakash Prasad
Department of Medical Oncology (Lab)
Dr BR Ambedkar Institute Rotary
	Cancer Hospital, All India Institute of
	Medical Sciences
New Delhi, India

Manuela Proietto
Oncology Unit, Oncology and
	Hematology Department
Piacenza General Hospital
Piacenza, Italy

S. M. Rezanur Rahman
Department of Pediatric Hematology
	and Oncology
Dhaka Medical College Hospital
Dhaka, Bangladesh

Amrita Rakesh
Department of Radiation Oncology
All India Institute of Medical Sciences
Patna, India

Daniel Gomez Ramos
Departments of Neurology
Mayo Clinic and Mayo Clinic
	Cancer Center
Phoenix, Arizona, USA

Rakesh Ranjan
Department of Radiation Oncology
All India Institute of Medical Sciences
Patna, India

Rohit Saini
Department of Radiation Oncology
All India Institute of Medical Sciences
Patna, India

Deepak Saini
Department of Materia Medica
State Lal Bahadur Shastri Homeopathic
	Medical College, and Hospital
Prayagraj, India

Abhishek Shankar
Department of Radiation Oncology
Dr Br Ambedkar Institute Rotary Cancer
	Hospital, All India Institute of
	Medical Sciences
Delhi, India

Arvind Kumar Shukla
School of Biomedical Convergence
	Engineering
Pusan National University, Yangsan,
	Gyeongsangnam-do
South Korea

Mayank Singh
Department of Medical Oncology
	(Lab)
Dr Br Ambedkar Institute Rotary Cancer
	Hospital, All India Institute of
	Medical Sciences
Delhi, India

Pritanjali Singh
Department of Radiation Oncology
All India Institute of Medical Sciences
Patna, India

Elisa Maria Stroppa
Oncology Unit, Oncology and
	Hematology Department
Piacenza General Hospital
Piacenza, Italy

Giulio Tarro
Emeritus Chief "D. Cotugno" Hospital,
	Naples-Italy, Chairman of the
	Committee on Biotechnologies
	and VirusSphere, WABT, Paris-
	France, Rector of the University
	Thomas More U.P.T.M., Rome-Italy,
	and President, Teresa & Luigi de
	Beaumont Bonelli Foundation for
	Cancer Research
Naples, Italy

Irene Testi
Oncology Unit, Oncology and
    Hematology Department
Piacenza General Hospital
Piacenza, Italy

Sonja Tomšič
Epidemiology and Cancer Registry
Institute of Oncology Ljubljana
Ljubljana, Slovenia

Aimen Vanood
Departments of Neurology
Mayo Clinic and Mayo Clinic
    Cancer Center
Phoenix, Arizona, USA

Vesna Zadnik
Epidemiology and Cancer Registry
Institute of Oncology Ljubljana
Ljubljana, Slovenia

Elena Zaffignani
Oncology Unit, Oncology and
    Hematology Department
Piacenza General Hospital
Piacenza, Italy

Tina Žagar
Epidemiology and Cancer Registry
Institute of Oncology Ljubljana
Ljubljana, Slovenia

Introduction

Giulio Tarro

The fear of other diseases, especially cancer, disappeared compared to the fear of contracting the COVID-19 virus. From 18 March 2020 to 8 May 2020, the death rate varied by 30.6% for COVID-19 with a cause of death of 92.5%. On the *Lancet Oncology* site the mortality rate was equal to 0.10 per subject between 40 and 49 years, while from leukemias to all other types of cancer (in particular, of the digestive tract, the mortality rate was 0.49 with an average age of 80 years). The characteristics of the cancer patient are given by 60% of subjects over 65 years; moreover diabetes and cardiovascular pathologies represent the most serious and critical complications, as for COVID-19. We are faced with patients who have an immunological deficit and therefore a greater risk of contagion and of developing various complications. A cancer diagnosis within the previous 5 years has been described in 20% of COVID-19 deaths. According to *Lancet Oncology* in 2020, a cancer patient transferred to a resuscitation unit for COVID-19 infection had a 4–5 times higher frequency of dying than patients without COVID-19. At this point, the Chinese experience becomes important, with the studies published in *Lancet Oncology* [1] concerning the city of Wuhan, the epicenter of the Chinese pandemic. We can note that what is described above is reported as a direct experience by Chinese colleagues, with regard to patients treated with chemotherapy or surgery before infection with COVID-19. In this scenario, patients with cancer or suspected cancer represent a challenge due to risk of death from untreated cancer versus serious complications from severe acute respiratory syndrome coronavirus 2 (SARS-CoV-2) [2–4].

This book aims to rise to meet the growing demand of practitioners, researchers, and educators for an introduction to key topics in the relationship between SARS-CoV-2 infection and cancers. In this regard, people affected by cancer or who are getting cancer treatment often are more susceptible to infections due to coexisting chronic diseases, overall poor health status, and systemic immunosuppressive states caused by both cancer and anticancer treatments. Different aspects of COVID-19 infection are considered in the chapters of this book:

- The many complications that have been reported by cancer patients due to COVID-19
- The use of telemedicine services for cancer patients during and after the COVID-19 pandemic
- How cancer diagnosis and management have been affected during the COVID-19 epidemic, based on the experiences in Slovenia and Italy
- Emerging challenges associated with different kinds of cancer (such as lung, colon, and brain)

DOI: 10.1201/9781003362562-1

- The clinical course, treatment efficacy, and risk factors in COVID-19 patients, as well as the direct and indirect risks of the global pandemic on the mortality of patients with cancer
- The dangerous possible synergy between pollution and COVID-19 on increasing male infertility and cancer in the near future with a great concern for health systems, especially in highly polluted areas of the world

Cancer patients have a higher risk of succumbing to COVID-19 due to immunosuppression, increased coexisting medical conditions, and, in cases of lung malignancy, underlying pulmonary compromise. Furthermore, patients with other types of cancer who are receiving active chemotherapy or immunotherapy may be particularly susceptible to this virus because of increased immunosuppression and/or dysfunction. In this context, decisions in oncology will become more complex since it is necessary to consider the heterogeneity of cancers and treatments as well as the heterogeneity of frailty levels among cancer patients.

This pandemic has raised new challenges in oncology, especially in the treatment and decision-making process in health-care organisations. This book will try to provide different data concerning COVID-19 in cancer patients to better manage decisions. Topics covered in this book are divided into different chapters on the management and eHealth process (telemedicine) for cancer patients. In this regard, this health crisis points out the need to change in the study of organisational models of care. Management models, protocols, and health procedures need to be updated and improved, and for this reason, a global strategy should be aimed at slowing down transmission of the virus to reduce mortality and morbidity. Specifically, the development of different systems of management for cancer patients needs new monitoring methods such as telemedicine and teleconsultations.

Furthermore, this book will focus on effect of COVID-19 on different types of cancer, while in the last chapter, the authors will describe the interaction among COVID-19, cancer, and pollution. The first chapter will provide a better understanding of the clinical course, treatment efficacy, and risk factors in COVID-19–positive cancer patients. In the second chapter, the authors will point out the difficulties in the complex care of cancer patients who require multidisciplinary approaches (such as with surgery, chemotherapy, targeted therapy, immunotherapy, and radiation) during this pandemic in Italy. In the third chapter, the authors will examine the current telemedicine landscape and challenges in cancer patients' care. This strategy can emerge not only as an interim solution, but it can be a valuable tool to deliver cancer care efficiently for a subset of patients intended to increase more and more in the future. In this regard, there are different concerns: the first is linked to limited access to the internet of poorer patients; and the second is the impossibility of carrying out an appropriate clinical examination from a distance, knowing that this routine clinical practice often reveals early signs which could lead to new investigations. In the fourth chapter, the authors will analyse and promptly report on how cancer diagnosis and management have been affected during the COVID-19 epidemic in Slovenia. The most substantial decrease in cancer diagnoses was recorded in April 2020, in the middle of the first COVID-19 wave. The overall cancer diagnoses burden was lower by about 30%, but there were some cancer types with a much larger drop (i.e. non-melanoma skin cancer by more than 60%). In autumn and winter, during the prolonged second wave, the decrease of cancer diagnoses was less prominent (10% for all cancer sites combined). Further, in the first wave there was a 33% and a 46% drop of first and control oncological referrals and 48%, 76%, and 42% less X-rays, mammograms, and ultrasounds performed at the IOL, respectively. The referrals as well as the diagnostic imaging were not affected significantly in the second wave; long-term studies are needed in order to evaluate what the effects of the perceived delay in diagnosis and treatment during the COVID-19 epidemic in Slovenia will be in terms of classical cancer burden indicators, such as poorer survival or a shift toward more advanced stage at diagnosis for specific cancer types. In the fifth chapter, the authors outline the clinical characteristics and outcome of children with cancer with SARS-CoV-2 infection in Dhaka Medical College Hospital, Bangladesh. Chapters 6, 7, and 8 deal with other topics regarding the effect of COVID-19 on different types of cancers (lung, brain, and colon). In Chapter 6, the authors will aim to explain their main priorities concerning COVID-19 infection in the scenario of lung cancer patients' group; patients with lung cancer need regular clinical and radiologic examinations and follow-ups, which might be hampered by the COVID-19 pandemic. Chapter 7 describes how the COVID-19 pandemic severely impacted access to care for patients affected by brain cancer; the authors discuss trends in neuro-oncologic care across the globe, focusing on changes in medical practice. In Chapter 8, the authors point out that some patients with severe COVID-19 can develop a dysbiotic microbiota of the gut and this impact might lead to increased incidence of colorectal cancer in the future or the aggravation of cancer symptoms in patients already afflicted, as reported by several studies. Chapter 9 points out that patients with cancer have longer SARS CoV-2 viral shedding compared with patients without cancer. Chapter 10 illustrates how the COVID-19 pandemic has revolutionised vaccine development. Many different approaches have been executed, including inactivated and live-attenuated virus, peptide and protein subunit vaccines, nucleic acid vaccines, and vaccines based on viral vectors. Specifically, the author will discuss the importance of vaccination for cancer patients since these patients infected with COVID-19 have poor outcomes, with an estimated mortality rate of 13% to 33%. Chapter 11 will focus on a dangerous possible synergy among pollution, COVID-19, and cancer. This issue could represent a great concern for health systems in the future, especially in highly polluted areas of the world.

Many studies have reported different results on the impact of cancer therapy on COVID-19 outcomes. Observational studies showed variable results regarding the impact of chemotherapy on COVID-19 outcomes [5–7]. For instance, two studies in China reported the increased risk of mortality in patients with COVID-19 under chemotherapy [8, 9]. In addition to the risk factors of patients with cancer who undergo chemotherapy, they are more susceptible to develop infections because of the suppression of their immune system [10]. Other studies did not find a significant association between severe COVID-19 and mortality in patients who had recently received chemotherapy [11]; for example, a large observational study from the U.S. Veterans Health Administration reported that there was no difference in mortality among those who received chemotherapy within 6 months of infection [12]. On the other hand, different cohort studies observed that cytotoxic chemotherapy was associated with poor outcomes [13–15]. In another registry study, the authors pointed out an increased risk of severe COVID-19 in patients who had received cytotoxic chemotherapy [16]. Immune checkpoint inhibitors (ICIs) are another therapy for cancer patients. Pneumonitis induced by these drugs can be correlated with dyspnea and/or other respiratory symptoms, and inflammatory lesions on chest after ICIs treatment, following exclusion of pulmonary infection, tumor progression, and other reasons. The incidence of pneumonitis in cancer patients during treatment was about 3%–5% [17]. Furthermore, ICIs could enhance the cytokine storm as seen in severe COVID-19, thus promoting poor outcomes of the infection in cancer patients [10]. Specifically, a retrospective study carried out from April 2020, found that the use of an ICIs within 90 days of COVID-19 diagnosis was a risk factor for hospitalization or severe disease. In this study, the authors found that the odds ratio for hospitalization was 2.52 (95% CI, 1.18–5.67; p = 0.013), and the HR (Heart Rate) for severe disease was 2.74 (95% CI, 1.37–5.46; p = 0.004) in multivariate models [18]. By contrast, in a first registry study conducted by the United Kingdom (UK) Coronavirus Cancer Monitoring Project through April 2020, the authors evaluated the impact of COVID-19 in 800 cancer patients treated with ICIs, but did not find association between use of ICIs and mortality rate [19]. In another French national study in June 2020, carried out on 1,289 patients with solid tumors and treated with ICIs within 4 weeks or 3 months, the authors did not report correlation between these drugs and mortality during the infection [20]. In another study, Fillmore et al. suggested an association between treatment type and outcome attributable to COVID-19 infection. In patients receiving ICIs within the last 6 months, COVID-19–attributable mortality (7.1%) was less than half in patients receiving chemotherapy (14.0%), hormone therapy (16.2%), or targeted therapy (14.1%), although statistical significance was not reached because of fewer observed deaths (7.1% in ICI vs 14.7% in not ICI; p = 0.53) [21]. In another analysis, Tan et al. showed that 228 cancer patients treated with ICIs had no higher risk of hospitalization or mortality than patients (patients 1,700) with similar cancers but treated with different therapies [22]. In an update from the UK Coronavirus Cancer Monitoring Project, the authors found that 2,515 cancer patients under treatment with ICIs had a decreased mortality rate (odds ratio, 0.52; 95% CI, p = 0.31–0.86) during the infection. They speculated that an antiviral T-cell immunity from ICIs in cancer patients could be induced during the infection or that cancer patients had a high survival due to antitumour effects [23]. Further studies on any association between ICIs and COVID-19 are necessary to better understand the T-cell exhaustion in patients with COVID-19 from the general population [24–27]. At the end, several meta-analyses on different data were performed to better evaluate whether exposure to ICIs was able to impact severe outcomes or mortality in patients with COVID-19 and cancer. In particular, Liu et al. studied many data from 19 papers with an ICI-treated group and a comparator group and reported no association between ICI treatment and mortality (odds ratio, 1.22; 95% CI, 0.91–1.62; p = 0.18) [28]. A few studies evaluated COVID-19 outcomes in cancer patients treated with specific lymphocyte-depleting therapies; B-cell depletion is associated with decreased antibody production, which is a risk factor for poor COVID-19 outcomes. There is limited information on COVID-19 outcomes in patients who have received CAR T-cell therapy targeting CD19, or B-cell maturation antigen. A recent European multicenter cohort study considered 56 patients who underwent CAR-T-cell therapy for B-cell-non-Hodgkin lymphoma (82.1%); most of them (62.5%) were in complete remission after CAR-T-cell therapy (62.5%) or had a partial response (12.5%). The median time from CAR-T-cell infusion to COVID-19 diagnosis was

7.4 months (min–max 1 day—25.3 months). Forty-five patients (80%) were admitted to hospital for COVID-19–related symptoms with a median duration of 25 days and 24 patients needed oxygen support (42.9%). Twenty-two (39.3%) patients were admitted to the intensive care unit (ICU) for a median duration of 14 days and 16 of these patients (72.7%) needed mechanical ventilation. Many different treatments were given but most patients received convalescent plasma, steroids, or remdesivir: 44.6% of them (25/56 patients) died and among these patients mortality could be attributed to COVID-19 in 41.1% (23/25 patients). This study identified age, poor performance status, multiple comorbidities, and active cancer diagnosis as key risk factors related to mortality [29].

Anti-CD20 monoclonal antibodies therapy, such as rituximab, is one of the most common drugs used to treat hematologic malignancies. Different studies on patients with hematologic malignancies, including lymphoma, found no association between COVID-19 outcomes and anti-CD20 therapies [30–34]. However, in a very small cohort study conducted on patients with hematologic malignancies, the authors reported 24.5% intensive care unit admission and 32.7% mortality [35]. Moreover, in another analysis from the UK Coronavirus Cancer Monitoring Project, the authors studied 877 patients with hematologic malignancies treated with anti-CD20 or anti-CD19 therapies but did not find an association with mortality. In the large National COVID Cohort Collaborative study, the authors found an increased risk for cancer patients treated with anti-CD20 agents [36]. Furthermore, different case reports described a chronic infection with SARS-CoV-2 in patients with lymphoma treated with different therapies (such as rituximab, hematopoietic stem cell transplant, or CAR T-cells) [37–43]. These cases could play a crucial role for evolution of SARS-CoV-2 in the host by creating mutational change and thus forming new variants of concern [44].

Today, cancer care has become difficult in European countries, especially in Italy where new diagnoses of cancer, according to the Italian Association of Medical Oncology, have decreased by 52%, while 64% of surgical interventions have suffered delays, both also linked to the fact that specific visits have been reduced by 57%. In this respect, management via telemedicine and the possibility of also carrying out a telematic clinic (obviously using telephone contact for correct information and the removal of any understandable doubts) should be maintained and enhanced. It is vitally important to translate lessons learned during the pandemic into effective policy and practice to guide health systems towards an equitable and person-centred digital future.

The therapeutic success in 60% of cancer patients still alive 5 years after the diagnosis of cancer is due to the success of considering cancer as a chronic disease with ample space for the use of drugs, multidisciplinarity, and geriatric and precision oncology. This experience has led to the maintenance of the patient's diagnosis and treatment programmes as a guideline, taking into account the multidisciplinary approach and the dignity of the patients themselves. In the context of epidemic control, it now becomes important to move from theory to practice with the knowledge already gained, in particular the use of monoclonal antibodies. This pandemic has taught us to consider the seriousness of the disease, especially when it affects oncological subjects, but also to have an attitude of hope, with the aim of carrying out updated study projects that allow for a better future for all.

REFERENCES

1. Mei H, Dong X, Wang Y, et al. Managing patients with cancer during the COVID-19 pandemic: Frontline experience from Wuhan. *Lancet Oncol* 2020;1(5):634–636. https://doi.org/10.1016/S1470-2045(20)30238-2X.

2. Yu J, Ouyang W, Chua MLK, Xie C. SARS-CoV-2 transmission in patients with cancer at a tertiary care hospital in Wuhan, China. *JAMA Oncol* 2020;6:1108. doi: 10.1001/jamaoncol.2020.0980.

3. Lewis MA. Between Scylla and Charybdis—oncologic decision making in the time of COVID-19. *N Engl J Med* 2020; 382:2285. doi: 10.1056/NEJMp2006588.

4. Hui D, Nortje N, George M, et al. Impact of an interdisciplinary goals-of-care program among medical inpatients at a comprehensive cancer center during the COVID-19 pandemic: A propensity score analysis. *J Clin Oncol* 2022;JCO2200849.

5. Dai M, Liu D, Liu M, et al: Patients with cancer appear more vulnerable to SARS-COV-2: A multi-center study during the COVID-19 outbreak. *Cancer Discov* 2020;10:783–791. doi: 10.1158/2159-8290.CD-20-0422.

6. Kuderer NM, Choueiri TK, Shah DP, et al. COVID-19 and cancer consortium clinical impact of COVID-19 on patients with cancer (CCC19): A cohort study. *Lancet* 2020;395:1907–1918 doi: 10.1016/S0140-6736(20)31187-9.

7. Clift AK, Coupland CAC, Keogh RH, et al. Living risk prediction algorithm (QCOVID) for risk of hospital admission and mortality from coronavirus 19 in adults: National derivation and validation cohort study. *BMJ* 2020;371:m3731. doi: 10.1136/bmj.m3731.

8. Tian J, Yuan X, Xiao J, et al. Clinical characteristics and risk factors associated with COVID-19 disease severity in patients with cancer in Wuhan, China: A multicentre, retrospective, cohort study. *Lancet Oncol* 2020;21:893–903. doi: 10.1016/S1470-2045(20)30309-0.

9. Yang K, Sheng Y, Huang C, et al. Clinical characteristics, outcomes, and risk factors for mortality in patients with cancer and COVID-19 in Hubei, China: A multicentre, retrospective, cohort study. *Lancet Oncol* 2020;21:904–913. doi: 10.1016/S1470-2045(20)30310-7.

10. Shams S, Mansoor K. COVID-19 and self-care measures by chemotherapy patients. *Asia-Pacific J Oncol Nurs* 2020;7:310. doi: 10.4103/apjon.apjon_20_20.

11. Lee LY, Cazier JB, Angelis V, et al. UK coronavirus monitoring project team; Kerr R, Middleton G. COVID-19 mortality in patients with cancer on chemotherapy or other anticancer treatments: A prospective cohort study. *Lancet* 2020;395(10241):1919–1926. doi: 10.1016/S0140-6736(20)31173-9.

12. Goyal P, Choi JJ, Pinheiro LC, et al. Clinical characteristics of COVID-19 in New York City. *N Engl J Med* 2020;382:2372–2374. doi: 10.1056/NEJMc2010419.

13. Cooksley CD, Avritscher EBC, Bekele BN, et al. Epidemiology and outcomes of serious influenza-related infections in the cancer population. *Cancer* 2005;104:618–628. doi: 10.1002/cncr.21203.

14. Henry BM, de Oliveira MHS, Benoit S, et al. Hematologic, biochemical and immune biomarker abnormalities associated with severe illness and mortality in coronavirus disease 2019 (COVID-19): A meta-analysis. *Clin Chem Lab Med* 2020;58:1021–1028. doi: 10.1515/cclm-2020-0369.

15. Qiu H, Wu J, Hong L, et al. Clinical and epidemiological features of 36 children with coronavirus disease 2019 (COVID-19) in Zhejiang, China: An observational cohort study. *Lancet Infect Dis* 2020;20:689–696. doi: 10.1016/S1473-3099(20)30198-5.

16. Grivas P, Khaki AR, Wise-Draper TM, et al. Association of clinical factors and recent anticancer therapy with COVID-19 severity among patients with cancer: A report from the COVID-19 and cancer consortium. *Ann Oncol* 2021;32(6):787–800. doi: 10.1016/j.annonc.2021.02.024.
17. Tiu BC, Zubiri L, Iheke J, et al. Real-world incidence and impact of pneumonitis in patients with lung cancer treated with immune checkpoint inhibitors: A multi-institutional cohort study. *J Immunother Cancer* 2022;10(6):e004670. doi: 10.1136/jitc-2022-004670.
18. Robilotti EV, Babady NE, Mead PA, et al. Determinants of COVID-19 disease severity in patients with cancer. *Nat Med* 2020;26(8):1218–1223. doi: 10.1038/s41591-020-0979-0.
19. UK Coronavirus Cancer Monitoring Project team. The UK coronavirus cancer monitoring project: Protecting patients with cancer in the era of COVID-19. *Lancet Oncol* 2020;21(5):622–624. doi: 10.1016/S1470-2045(20)30230-8.
20. Goldman JD, Gonzalez MA, Rüthrich MM, et al. COVID-19 and cancer: Special considerations for patients receiving immunotherapy and immunosuppressive cancer therapies. *Soc Clin Oncol Educ Book* 2022;42:76–188.
21. Fillmore NR, La J, Szalat RE, et al. Prevalence and outcome of COVID-19 infection in cancer patients: A national veterans affairs study. *J Natl Cancer Inst* 2021;113(6):691–698. doi: 10.1093/jnci/djaa159.
22. Tan R, Yun C, Seetasith A, et al. Impact of immune checkpoint inhibitors on COVID-19 severity in patients with cancer. *Oncologist* 2022;27:236–243. doi: 10.1093/oncolo/oyab083.
23. Várnai C, Palles C, Arnold R, et al. UKCCMP team. Mortality among adults with cancer undergoing chemotherapy or immunotherapy and infected with COVID-19. *JAMA Netw Open* 2022;5:e220130. doi: 10.1001/jamanetworkopen.2022.0130.
24. Su Y, Chen D, Yuan D, et al. ISB-Swedish COVID19 biobanking unit. Multi-omics resolves a sharp disease-state shift between mild and moderate COVID-19. *Cell* 2020;183:1479–1495. doi: 10.1016/j.cell.2020.10.037.
25. Mathew D, Giles JR, Baxter AE, et al. Deep immune profiling of COVID-19 patients reveals distinct immunotypes with therapeutic implications. *Science* 2020;369:eabc8511. 26. doi: 10.1126/science.abc8511.
26. De Biasi S, Meschiari M, Gibellini L, et al. Marked T cell activation, senescence, exhaustion and skewing towards TH17 in patients with COVID-19 pneumonia. *Nat Commun* 2020;11:3434. 27. doi: 10.1038/s41467-020-17292-4.
27. Rha MS, Shin EC. Activation or exhaustion of CD8+ T cells in patients with COVID-19. *Cell Mol Immunol* 2021;18:2325–2333. doi: 10.1038/s41423-021-00750-4.
28. Liu Y, Liu S, Qin Y, et al. Does prior exposure to immune checkpoint inhibitors treatment affect incidence and mortality of COVID-19 among the cancer patients: The systematic review and meta-analysis. *Int Immunopharmacol* 2021;101:108242. doi: 10.1016/j.intimp.2021.108242.
29. Spanjaart AM, Ljungman P, de La Camara R, et al. Poor outcome of patients with COVID-19 after CAR T-cell therapy for B-cell malignancies: Results of a multicenter study on behalf of the European Society for Blood and Marrow Transplantation (EBMT) Infectious Diseases Working Party and the European Hematology Association (EHA) Lymphoma Group. *Leukemia* 2021;35:3585–3588. doi: 10.1038/s41375-021-01466-0.
30. Malard F, Genthon A, Brissot E, et al. COVID-19 outcomes in patients with hematologic disease. *Bone Marrow Transplant* 2020;55:2180–2184. doi: 10.1038/s41409-020-0931-4.

31. Wood WA, Neuberg DS, Thompson JC, et al. Outcomes of patients with hematologic malignancies and COVID-19: A report from the ASH research collaborative data Hub. *Blood Adv* 2020;4:5966–5975. doi: 10.1182/bloodadvances.2020003170.
32. Martın-Moro F, Marquet J, Piris M, et al. Survival study of hospitalised patients with concurrent COVID-19 and haematological malignancies. *Br J Haematol* 2020;190:e16–e20. doi: 10.1111/bjh.16801.
33. He W, Chen L, Chen L, et al. COVID-19 in persons with haematological cancers. *Leukemia* 2020;34:1637–1645. doi: 10.1038/s41375-020-0836-7.
34. Vijenthira A, Gong IY, Fox TA, et al. Outcomes of patients with hematologic malignancies and COVID-19: A systematic review and meta-analysis of 3377 patients. *Blood* 2020;136:2881–2892. doi: 10.1182/blood.2020008824.
35. Levavi H, Lancman G, Gabrilove J. Impact of rituximab on COVID-19 outcomes. *Ann Hematol* 2021;100:2805–2812. doi: 10.1007/s00277-021-04662-1.
36. Andersen KM, Bates BA, Rashidi ES, et al. National COVID cohort collaborative consortium. Long-term use of immunosuppressive medicines and in-hospital COVID-19 outcomes: A retrospective cohort study using data from the National COVID Cohort Collaborative. *Lancet Rheumatol* 2022;4:e33–e41. doi: 10.1016/S2665-9913(21)00325-8.
37. Aydillo T, Gonzalez-Reiche AS, Aslam S, et al. Shedding of viable SARS-CoV-2 after immunosuppressive therapy for cancer. *N Engl J Med* 2020;383:2586–2588. doi: 10.1056/NEJMc2031670.
38. Avanzato VA, Matson MJ, Seifert SN, et al. Case study: Prolonged infectious SARS-CoV-2 shedding from an asymptomatic immunocompromised individual with cancer. *Cell.* 2020;183:1901–1912.e9. doi:10.1016/j.cell.2020.10.049.
39. Baang JH, Smith C, Mirabelli C, et al. Prolonged severe acute respiratory syndrome coronavirus 2 replication in an immunocompromised patient. *J Infect Dis* 2021;223:23–27. doi: 10.1093/infdis/jiaa666.
40. Kemp SA, Collier DA, Datir RP, et al. COVID-19 genomics UK (COG-UK) consortium. SARS-CoV-2 evolution during treatment of chronic infection. *Nature* 2021;592:277–282. doi: 10.1038/s41586-021-03291-y.
41. Khatamzas E, Antwerpen MH, Rehn A, et al. Accumulation of mutations in antibody and CD8 T cell epitopes in a B cell depleted lymphoma patient with chronic SARS-CoV-2 infection. *Nat Commun* 2022;13:5586. doi.10.1038/s41467-022-32772-5.
42. Nussenblatt V, Roder AE, Das S, et al. Year-long COVID-19 infection reveals within-host evolution of SARS-CoV-2 in a patient with B-cell depletion. *J Infect Dis* 2022;225:1118–1123. doi: 10.1093/infdis/jiab622.
43. Truong TT, Ryutov A, Pandey U, et al. Increased viral variants in children and young adults with impaired humoral immunity and persistent SARS-CoV-2 infection: A consecutive case series. *EBioMedicine* 2021;67:103355. doi: 10.1016/j.ebiom.2021.103355.
44. Corey L, Beyrer C, Cohen MS, et al. SARS-CoV-2 variants in patients with immunosuppression. *N Engl J Med* 2021;385:562–566. doi: 10.1056/NEJMsb2104756.

1

Management of Cancer Patients during the COVID-19 Pandemic

Luigi Cavanna, Chiara Citterio, Elena Zaffignani, Massimo Ambroggi, and Gabriele Cremona

Introduction

A novel coronavirus named severe acute respiratory syndrome coronavirus 2 (SARS-CoV-2) emerged in Wuhan, China in December 2019, and has quickly spread globally [1–3].

The World Health Organization (WHO) ruled coronavirus disease 2019 (COVID-19), caused by SARS-CoV-2, to be a public health emergency of international concern and declared a pandemic [3]. Cancer patients are at high risk of acquiring COVID-19 because of poor general health and their systemic immunosuppressive state caused by the cancer and/or anticancer treatments such as chemotherapy, radiation, surgery, and steroids. In addition, cancer patients have frequently scheduled visits to hospital and clinics, which can increase the risk of catching COVID-19 [4–7]. As reported initially from China, patients with cancer have a markedly elevated risk of intubation, intensive care unit admission, or death, both for cancer patients receiving active anticancer treatment and cancer survivors [8].

Cancer Patients during the COVID-19 Pandemic and their Management

Patients with cancer are generally presumed to have a major risk of developing infectious complications; consequently, control measures of COVID-19 transmission are very important. After China, Europe was affected next by a sudden surge of cases and Italy was the first country to be affected severely. By 1 April, within a month of the first case that was reported in the Lombardy region in northern Italy, 100,000 cases and more than 12,000 deaths had been reported in the country [9]. Out of 909 patients who died in the hospital in that registry, 150 patients had active cancer within the last 5 years [10]. The Lombardy region was the epicenter of the pandemic and accounted for 63.5% deaths across the country. Our group reported the first 25 cancer patients [11] in a western country (Italy) in a district very near (10 minutes by car) to the epicenter of the outbreak of COVID-19 in Italy, and the catastrophic nature of the Lombardy outbreak has been widely publicised [12]. All of these 25 cancer patients were diagnosed with laboratory-confirmed SARS-COV-2 infection, with reverse transcription poly-merase chain reaction in nasal-pharyngeal swabs, which caused the respiratory illness COVID-19, defined as an oxygen saturation (SaO2) of 94% or less while they were breathing ambient air, or a ratio of the partial pressure of oxygen (PaO2) to the fraction of inspired oxygen (FiO2) of less than 300 mmHg [13]. A total of 13 cases (52%) had a history of smoking for more than 20 years. The majority of patients, 19 (76%), had several comorbidities (in particular diabetes mellitus [32%], hypertension [64%] and chronic obstructive pulmonary disease [28%]). Many oncologic patients coming from the epicenter of the outbreak of COVID-19 were actively receiving treatment at the oncologic department of the hospital of Piacenza. In this series of 25 cancer patients with COVID-19, nine (36%) are dead compared with 16 (13%) dead patients with COVID-19 without cancer. The majority of the 25 cancer patients (76%) showed meta-static disease, and unfavorable prognostic factors were advanced age (mean 74.44 ± 7.21 years for dead patients versus 68.38 ± 10.16 years for alive patients) and comorbidities.

Trapani et al [14] reported outcomes from a small case series of nine cancer patients with lab-confirmed COVID-19 who were referred to the European Institute of Oncology in the Lombardy region. Three were inpatients and six were treated as outpatients. No cancer type was predominant. Eight of the nine patients were actively receiving cancer therapy ($n = 4$ chemotherapy, $n = 2$ immunotherapy, and $n = 2$ small molecules). Three were being treated with curative intent and five patients had meta-static disease. None of the patients required ICU admission, no deaths were reported, and all three inpatients were discharged. In United Kingdom Coronavirus Cancer Monitoring Project (UKCCMP) generated database from prospective cohort of 800 patients across 55 cancer centers in the country [15]. Gastrointestinal, respiratory, breast, male genital, and haematological cancers were the most common types (10% or more). Forty-three percent of patients had metastatic disease. Sixty-five patients had received some form of cancer treatment within the last 4 weeks. More than half of the patients receiving treatment had received cytotoxic chemotherapy. Forty-five patients had severe or critical infection. Mortality rate was high at 28% (226 out of 800) with 93% of those deaths due to COVID-19. Patients who died, as in our reports [11, 16], had higher number of co-morbidities and were older than those who sur-vived. Interestingly, patients who had recently received chemotherapy (within 4 weeks of COVID-19 infection) did not have increased mortality as compared to those who did not receive chemotherapy. In the United States, New York City became the epicen-ter of the pandemic soon after [17]. Mehta V et al [18] have reported outcomes from a New York City hospital on 218 cancer patients with COVID-19. Seventy-five patients had solid tumours and 25% had haematological malignancies. Most common tumour type was genitourinary ($n = 46$) followed by breast ($n = 28$) and colorectal cancer ($n = 21$). A total of 61 (28%) patients died. Mortality rate was higher than 50% in patients with lung (55%) and pancreatic cancer (67%). Breast and genitourinary cancer were associated with a relatively lower mortality rate (14% and 15% respectively). Among haematological malignancies, myeloid neoplasm had a higher mortality rate than lym-phoid tumours. COVID-19 and Cancer Consortium (CCC19) reported outcomes of 928 cancer patients with COVID-19 infection from the United States, Canada, and Spain [19]. The most common tumour type was breast cancer ($n = 191$) followed by prostate cancer ($n = 152$). Of patients, 654 had solid tumours, 167 had haematological malignancies, and 107 had multiple cancers. Forty-five patients were reported to be in remission and 43% had active cancer. Among those with active cancer, 74% had stable or responding cancer, and 26% had progressive cancer. Out of 366 patients on active treatment, 160 received chemotherapy in the last 4 weeks and 206 patients underwent other forms of cancer therapy. Before the COVID-19 vaccine's availability, the importance of widespread SARS-COV-2 testing as a strategy to facilitate early diagnosis of COVID-19, allowing adequate measures of containment of the pandemic, and maintain the appropriate therapeutic pathway for patients with cancer has been reported [20]. In this context our group reported the prevalence of COVID-19 infection in asymptomatic cancer patients in a district with high prevalence of SARS-CoV-2 in Italy [21] and in this report from April 2020 to June 2020, in a 2-month period, 260 consecutive, asymptomatic (for COVID-19) cancer patients were tested for COVID-19. There were 160 women and 100 men; 218 patients were under active anticancer treatment, 32 in the diagnostic/staging phase waiting for treatment, and 10 treated with supportive care only. Ten of the 260 patients (3.85%) showed COVID-19 positivity. Our data indicate a high prevalence of COVID-19 in cancer patients in an area with a high prevalence of SARS-CoV-2 infection. That routine COVID-19 testing of cancer patients when asymptomatic allowed an early detection, isolation, and treatment, avoiding viral spread among other frail patients and among medical/nurse staff. It must be emphasised that the major oncologic associations – American Society of Clinical Oncology (ASCO), European Society for Medical Oncology (ESMO), Associazione Italiana di Oncologia Medica (AIOM), Collegio degli Oncologi Medici Universitari (COMU), and Collegio Italiano dei Primari Oncologi Medici Ospedalieri (CIPOMO) – have rapidly produced guidance on decisions about management of patients with cancer during the COVID-19 crisis. In this extraordinary period many efforts have been made by governments, the oncology community, and caregivers to protect frail cancer patients from COVID-19 infection [22–26]. In this scenario, cancer patients must receive priority that they have gone without for so long. The challenge is difficult, but it will be fundamental to adopt strategies to support the cancer patients who need care. The cancer programmes will need to encompass the care model, operational requirements, financial implications, and near- and long-term strategic considerations. For people in the best of circumstances, the pandemic has been a stressful and trying time. For cancer patients, it has been a physical and emotional ordeal.

REFERENCES

1. Lu R, Zhao X, Li J. et al. Genomic characterization and epidemiology of 2019 novel coronavirus: Implications for virus origins and receptor binding. *Lancet* 2020;395(10224):565–574.
2. Wu Z, McGoogan JM. Characteristics of and important lessons from the coronavirus disease 2019 (COVID-19) outbreak in China: Summary of a report of 72? 314 cases from the Chinese Center for Disease Control and Prevention. *JAMA* 2020;323(13):1239–1242.
3. World Health Organization. Coronavirus disease (COVID-19) outbreak (2020). www.who.int/dg/speeches/detail/who-director-general-s-opening-remarks-at-the-media-briefing-on-covid-19---11-march-2020.
4. Kamboj M, Sepkowitz KA. Nosocomial infections in patients with cancer. *Lancet Oncol* 2009;10(6):589–597.
5. Li JY, Duan XF, Wang LP. et al. Selective depletion of regulatory T cell subsets by docetaxel treatment in patients with non-small-cell lung cancer. *J Immunol Res* 2014;2014:286170.

6. Longbottom ER, Torrance HD, Owen HC. et al. Features of postoperative immune suppression are reversible with interferon gamma and independent of interleukin-6 pathways. *Ann Surg* 2016;264(2):370–377.

7. Sica A, Massarotti M. Myeloid suppressor cells in cancer and autoimmunity. *J Autoimmun* 2017;85:117–125.

8. Liang W, Guan W, Chen R. et al. Cancer patients in SARS-CoV-2 infection: A nationwide analysis in China. *Lancet Oncol* 2020;21(3):335–337.

9. Fratino L, Procopio G, Di Maio M, Cinieri S, Leo S, Beretta G. Coronavirus: Older persons with cancer in Italy in the COVID19 pandemic. *Front Oncol* 2020;10:648.

10. Instituto Superiore di Sanità. Characteristics of COVID-19 patients dying in Italy. Report based on available data on 30 March 2020.

11. Stroppa EM, Toscani I, Citterio C, Anselmi E, Zaffignani E, Codeluppi M, Cavanna L. Coronavirus disease-2019 in cancer patients. A report of the first 25 cancer patients in a western country (Italy). *Future Oncol* 2020 July;16(20):1425–1432.

12. Horowitz J. Italy's healthcare system groans under coronavirus- a warning to the world. New York Times; (2020). www.nytimes.com/2020/03/12/world/europe/12italy-coronavirus-health-care.html.

13. Time. The Italian doctor flattening the curve by treating COVID-19 patients in their homes (2020). http://time.com/5816874/italy-coronavirus-patients-treating-home/.

14. Trapani D, Marra A. Giuseppe Curigliano the experience on coronavirus disease 2019 and cancer from oncology hub institution in Milan, Lombardy region. *Eur J Cancer* 2020;132:199–206.

15. Lee LYW, Cazier JB, Starkey T, Turnbull CD. UK coronavirus cancer monitoring project team, Rachel Kerr, Gary Middleton COVID-19 mortality in patients with cancer on chemotherapy or other anticancer treatments: A prospective cohort study. *Lancet* 2020;395:1919–1926.

16. Cavanna L, Citterio C, Toscani I, Franco C, Magnacavallo A, Caprioli S, Cattadori E, Nunzio CD, Pane R, Schiavo R, Biasini C, Ambroggi M. Cancer patients with COVID-19: A retrospective study of 51 patients in the district of Piacenza, Northern Italy. *Future Sci OA* 2020 November 24;7(1):FSO645.

17. John Hopkins University coronavirus resource center. https://coronavirus.jhu.edu/map.html.

18. Mehta V, Goel S, Verma A, et al. Case fatality rate of cancer patients with COVID-19 in a New York Hospital system. *Cancer Discov* 2020;10(7):935–941. Published Online First 1 May.

19. Kuderer NM, Choueiri TK, Shah DP, et al. Clinical impact of COVID-19 on patients with cancer (CCC19): A cohort study. *Lancet* 2020;395:1907–1918.

20. OnCovid Study Group, Pinato DJ, Patel M, Scotti L, Colomba E, Dolly S, et al. Time-dependent COVID-19 mortality in patients with cancer: An updated analysis of the OnCovid registry. *JAMA Oncol* 2022 January 1;8(1):114–122. doi: 10.1001/jamaoncol.2021.6199.

21. Cavanna L, Citterio C, Di Nunzio C, Biasini C, Palladino MA, Ambroggi M, Madaro S, Bidin L, Porzio R, Proietto M. Prevalence of COVID-19 infection in asymptomatic cancer patients in a district with high prevalence of SARS-CoV-2 in Italy. *Cureus* 2021 Mar 9;13(3):e13774.

22. Kutikov A, Weinberg DS, Edelman MJ, Horwitz EM, Uzzo RG, Fisher RI. A war on two fronts: Cancer care in the time of COVID-19. *Ann Intern Med* 2020 June 2;172(11):756–758. doi: 10.7326/M20-1133.

23. Lewis MA. Between Scylla and Charybdis – oncologic decision making in the time of Covid-19. *N Engl J Med* 2020 January 11;382(24):2285–2287.

24. AIOM, CIPOMO, COMU. RISCHIO INFETTIVO DA CORONAVIRUS COVID 19: INDICAZIONI PER L'ONCOLOGIA. March 2020. https://www.aiom.it/wp-content/uploads/2020/03/20200313_COVID-19_indicazioni_AIOM-CIPOMO-COMU.pdf.

25. ASCO Special Report: Guide to cancer care delivery during the COVID-19 pandemic. 19 May 2020. https://old-prod.asco.org/sites/new-www.asco.org/files/content-files/2020-ASCO-Guide-Cancer-COVID19.pdf.

26. European Society for Medical Oncology: Cancer patient management during the COVID-19 pandemic. 2020. https://www.esmo.org/guidelines/cancer-patient-management-during-the-covid-19-pandemic Google Scholar.

2

The COVID-19 Impact and Cancer Care in Italy: A Case Study

Luigi Cavanna, Chiara Citterio, Camilla Di Nunzio, Claudia Biasini,
Nicola Inzerilli, Elena Orlandi, Manuela Proietto, Irene Testi,
and Monica Muroni

Introduction

Severe acute respiratory syndrome coronavirus 2 (SARS-Cov-2) respiratory disease, coronavirus disease 2019 (COVID-19), has been spreading worldwide, changing everyday life. Cancer patients are at high risk of acquiring this virus owing to poor general conditions, systemic immunosuppressive state caused by the cancer itself, and/or anticancer treatments such as chemotherapy, radiation, surgery, and steroids. In addition, cancer patients have frequent scheduled visits to the hospital and clinics, which can increase the risk of catching COVID-19 [1].

As reported initially from China, patients with cancer have a markedly elevated risk of intubation, intensive care unit admission, or death, both for cancer patients receiving active anticancer treatment and cancer survivors [2]. In oncological units in Italy, clinical consultations for patients not requiring active treatment for cancer and follow-up were performed at wider intervals of time [3–5], and according to Italian oncologists, other types of preventive measures have been established to reduce virus spread; patients are subjected to a triage before admission to the hospital, and more specifically, the triage screening tools used include phone calls, virtual consultations, and telemedicine [6, 7].

The COVID-19 Impact and Cancer Care in Italy: A Case Study

In Italy, following the Chinese model, containment measures to reduce the risk of COVID-19 spread were promptly activated. The Italian government has implemented extraordinary measures to restrict the spread of the virus, and the first national decree, issued on 8 March 2020, instituted a containment zone concerning the most affected areas of the country, called the red zone, which at that time included three regions of north Italy: Emilia Romagna, Lombardy, and Veneto. In this extraordinary and dramatic context, the Italian college of directors of the National Health

DOI: 10.1201/9781003362562-3

System (NHS) of the Hospital Department of Medical Oncology (Collegio Italiano Primary Oncologi Medici Ospedalieri [CIPOMO]) promoted a survey during the first COVID-19 wave, aiming to evaluate the impact of COVID-19 on clinical activity of oncologists and the implementation of containment measures of COVID-19 spread. This survey was launched online on 12 March 2020, and closed on 15 March 2020. Results of this survey have been published [6]. Briefly, 122 head physicians of oncology units participated in this national survey: measures to reduce hospital access for oncologic patients were taken almost throughout the country, delaying visits when possible for patients not urgent, triage of patients before entering the hospital, preventive isolation, and diagnostic procedures applied for patients with suspected infection of COVID-19. For visitors and caregivers, access to inpatient and outpatient clinic was prohibited, and anticancer treatment was ensured when necessary and not delayed for cancer patients with aggressive tumors. During the second wave of COVID-19, the CIPOMO promoted another Italian national survey to evaluate the impact of COVID-19 on oncologists' clinical activity and the changes from the first COVID-19 pandemic wave [8]. This second national survey showed a better organisation of clinical activities with regular testing among healthcare practitioners with better protection of cancer patients. A dramatic decline in access to screening programmes was registered; it must be emphasised that in Italy are active three screening programmes for uterus (cervical), breast, and colorectal cancer. In 2020, a national Italian survey was performed by the National Centre for Screening Monitoring (ONS) [9]. The results of the survey showed that screening tests for breast, colorectal, and cervical cancer decreased by 37.6%, 45.5%, and 43.4% in 2020, compared with 2019. The estimated numbers of undiagnosed lesions were 3,324 for breast cancer, 1,299 for colorectal cancer, 7,474 colorectal advanced adenomas, and 2,782 CNN2 or more severe cervical lesions [9]. Moving from the national to a regional survey during the first COVID-19 wave, Brandes A. et al [7] performed a multidomain survey focused on patients, health-care workers, risk reduction measures, and clinical trials in all the medical oncology departments from the Italian Emilia Romagna Region. This survey showed that the measures applied to patients and health workers partially converged in all the departments while major divergences were found in the clinical trials domain. High rate of COVID-19 infections occurred among medical doctors (21/208, 10.1%), while the rate of infection among nurses was 5.7% (24/418) [7]. Moving to a provincial territory analysis, Ambroggi M et al [10] reported the impact of the COVID-19 pandemic on the oncologic activities (diagnosis, treatment, clinical trials enrollment) of a general hospital in a district with high prevalence of SARS-COV-2 in Italy. The authors retrospectively analysed the data during the first wave of oncologic activity, namely new cancer diagnosis, types of treatment (intravenous or by mouth), clinical research studies, and drug utilisation, and compared the findings with those of 2019, before the pandemic. This study was performed in the district of Piacenza, North Italy. In 2020, a significant reduction in new cancer diagnoses was demonstrated when compared with 2019, with 17.4% fewer cancer diagnoses, 84.5% fewer patients enrolled in clinical trials, a 10.6% reduction in intravenous antitumor treatment, and a 42.7% increase in oral anticancer treatment. These data suggest that the COVID-19 pandemic had a deep impact on the real-world management of cancer patients in a district of Italy with a high prevalence of COVID-19 [10].

In conclusion, the COVID-19 pandemic has heavily affected cancer care: patients, caregivers, medical oncologists, nurses, and social care workers in oncology, with negative fallout in preclinical, clinical, and translational research. Now all the actors of the sanitary system should establish a strong alliance to make up for lost time due to the COVID-19 pandemic, allowing for better care for cancer patients [11–13].

The new challenges for the Italian Ministry of Health, the national government, and the regions are (1) sustainable funding of the National Health System, (2) to reorganise the National Health System by providing and strengthening health care services (e.g. prevention/public health, primary/community care), and in addition, (3) to increase the workforce in the medium and long term, to modernise the physical infrastructures of the health care system; all the while keeping in mind that reinforcing the country's preparedness to future epidemics can no longer be postponed.

REFERENCES

1. El Saghir NS. Oncology care and education during the coronavirus (COVID-19) pandemic. AsCO Connection. 19 March 2020. https://connection.asco.org/blogs/oncology-care-and-education-during-coronavirus-covid-19-pandemic.
2. Liang W, Guan W, Chen R. et al. Cancer patients in SARS-CoV-2 infection: A nationwide analysis in China. *Lancet Oncol* 21, 335–337 (2020).
3. National Cancer Institute. Coronavirus guidance. Updated 1 April 2020. Accessed 9 April 2020. https://ctep.cancer.gov/investigatorResources/corona_virus_guidance.htm.
4. European Medicines Agency. Guidance on the management of clinical trials during the COVID-19 (coronavirus) pandemic (version 3, 28 April 2020) (2020). https://ec.europa.eu/health/sites/health/files/files/eudralex/vol-10/guidanceclinicaltrials_covid19_en.pdf.
5. European Society for Medical Oncology: Cancer patient management during the COVID-19 pandemic. 2020. https://www.esmo.org/guidelines/cancer-patient-management-during-the-covid-19-pandemic.
6. Indini A, Aschele C, Cavanna L. et al. Reorganisation of medical oncology departments during the novel coronavirus disease-19 pandemic: A nationwide Italian survey. *Eur J Cancer* 2020;132:17–23.
7. Brandes AA, Ardizzoni A, Artioli F. et al. Fighting cancer in coronavirus disease era: Organization of work in medical oncology departments in Emilia Romagna region of Italy. *Future Oncol* 2020;16(20):1433–1439.
8. Indini A, Pinotti G, Artioli F. et al. Management of patients with cancer during the COVID-19 pandemic: The Italian perspective on second wave. *Eur J Cancer* 2021;148:112–116.
9. Battisti F, Falini P, Gorini G. et al. Cancer screening programmes in Italy during the COVID-19 pandemic: An updated of a nationwide survey on activity volumes and delayed diagnoses. *Ann Ist Super Sanità* 2022;58(1):16–24.
10. Ambroggi M, Citterio C, Vecchia S. et al. Impact of the COVID-19 pandemic on the oncologic activities (diagnosis, treatment, clinical trials enrollment) of a general hospital in a district with high prevalence of SARS-COV-2 in Italy. *Support Care Cancer* 2022;30:3225–3231.
11. Cavanna L. Equità di accesso alle cure in oncologia. I Liberati's principles per una nuova governance della ricerca. Recenti Prog In *Medicina* 2022;113(10):622. doi: 10.1701/3888.38709.

12. Grassi O, Oleari F, Citterio C, et al. Home care: Home venous access device insertion during COVID-19 pandemic in not autonomous patients. From an emergency activity to a daily work practice. *Recenti Prog In Medicina* 2022;13(11):669–673. doi: 10.1701/3907.38894.
13. Beretta GD, Casolino R, Corsi DC et al. Position paper of the Italian Association of Medical Oncology on the impact of COVID-19 on Italian oncology and the path forward: The 2021 Matera statement. *ESMO Opne* 2022;7:4. https://doi.org/10.1016/j.esmoop.2022.100538.

3

The Importance of Telemedicine for Cancer Patients during the COVID-19 Pandemic: Perspective and Challenge

Luigi Cavanna, Chiara Citterio, Camilla Di Nunzio, Elisa Anselmi, Elena Zaffignani, Giulia Claire Giudice, and Nicoletta Bacchetta

Introduction

A novel coronavirus named severe acute respiratory syndrome coronavirus 2 (SARS-CoV-2) emerged in Wuhan, China in December 2019, and has quickly spread globally [1–3]. Patients with cancer are generally presumed to have a major risk of developing infectious complications. Consequently, control measures of COVID-19 transmission are very important. Cancer patients are at high risk of acquiring this virus because of poor general conditions, a systemic immunosuppressive state caused by cancer itself, and/or anticancer treatment such as chemotherapy, radiation, surgery, steroids, etc. In addition, cancer patients have frequently scheduled visits to hospitals and clinics that can increase the risk of catching coronavirus disease 2019 (COVID-19) [4, 5]. As previously reported from China, patients with cancer have a markedly elevated risk of intensive care unit (ICU) admission, intubation, or death, both for cancer patients receiving active anticancer treatment and cancer survivors [6]. So oncologic practices have changed in response to the SARS-CoV-2 pandemic; when possible, oncologists postponed chemotherapy treatments, as well as surgery; also radiotherapy was abbreviated and some treatments were switched from intravenous to oral therapies. In the oncological units in Italy, clinical consultations for patients who didn't require active treatment for cancer and follow-up were done at wider intervals of time [7–9].

The Importance of Telemedicine for Cancer Patients during the COVID-19 Pandemic

During the COVID-19 Pandemic oncologic patients and caregivers were subjected to triage before admission to the hospital, and more specifically, the triage screening tools used were phone calls, virtual consultations, and telemedicine [9, 10]. A systematic review and meta-synthesis of qualitative literature on the use of telemedicine in cancer care during the COVID-19 pandemic has been reported from Iran [11]. In this research 19 studies were included in the final meta-synthesis that concerned 684

DOI: 10.1201/9781003362562-4

health-care providers, 256 patients, 16 caregivers, and 1 patient advocate. Health-care providers included leaders of cancer centres, home care professionals, social workers, nurses, physicians, care managers, pharmacists, psychologists, and other professionals in the oncology field. This meta-synthesis highlighted that telemedicine was more effective in managing cancer patients' primary health-care needs and follow up visits; in addition it contributed to recognise advantages, disadvantages, prerequisites, and preferences of patients and providers based on their lived experience [11]. A systematic review of the literature on telehealth in urology including 11 studies concerning prostate cancer was performed by Novara et al [12]. In this review it was demonstrated that time in minutes devoted to patient care in video visits showed no difference with standard visit time. Telemedicine during the COVID-19 pandemic was rapidly incorporated at the oncology division of Tel Aviv Medical Center and a survey was done among adult patients with cancer treated there between March and May 2020 [13]. The results of this survey showed that 232 patients used a telemedicine platform between March and May 2020, and 172 (74%) agreed to participate in the survey. Family members/caregivers were commonly present during telemedicine meetings. It is very important to make evident that in this study a multivariate analysis revealed that higher satisfaction and visits for routine surveillance were both predictors of willingness to continue future telemedicine meetings over physical encounters and telemedicine was perceived as safe and effective. A systematic review on management of cancer patients during the COVID-19 pandemic using telemedicine was done by Salehi F. et al [14]; 2614 articles were retrieved after searching the database, of them 305 studies were eligible for further full-text review and finally only 16 articles were selected for the final analysis. The results of this review indicated that the virtual visit service was the most common telemedicine service used during the COVID-19 pandemic. The authors of the review concluded that telemedicine can provide continued access to necessary health service in oncology care and showed an important role during the COVID-19 pandemic [14]. A study from France [15], based on qualitative method with semi-directed interviews with doctors from the oncology and supportive care departments of Foch Hospital who had used telemedicine during the first wave of the COVID-19 pandemic, showed a large difference between doctors in terms of their views concerning telemedicine before and after the first wave of the COVID-19 pandemic in France [15]. However, during the COVID-19 pandemic many providers and patients had to adopt the use of telemedicine in a relatively short time, and it was hypothesised that socioeconomic differences could create gaps in telemedicine adoption among different patient groups during this extraordinary and dramatic period [16]. Luo J et al [16] from the United States demonstrated that patients who used video visits were younger (median age 48.12) and more likely to be white and have private insurance, while patients who used telephone visits were older (median age 57–58) and more likely to be black and have public insurance. This study revealed potential inequities and disparities in telemedicine adoption. In conclusion, telemedicine provided important solutions for cancer patients during the COVID-19 pandemic and it should be implemented in the future. However, providers and clinicians should avoid the risk that telemedicine remains relegated to a small minority of cancer patients [17] and the risk of potential inequities in telemedicine adoption [17, 18]. In summary, understanding barriers to telemedicine use and preferred modalities of communication among different populations can play a crucial role in interventions at different socioecological levels to ensure the continued evolution of telemedicine is equitable.

REFERENCES

1. Lu R, Zhao X, Li J, et al. Genomic characterization and epidemiology of 2019 novel coronavirus: Implications for virus origins and receptor binding. *Lancet* 2020;395:565–574. doi:10.1016/S0140-6736(20)30251-8.
2. Wu Z, McGoogan JM. Characteristics of and important lessons from the coronavirus disease 2019 outbreak in China: Summary of a report of 72,314 cases from the Chinese Center for Disease Control and Prevention. *JAMA* 2020;323:1239–1242. doi:10.1001/jama.2020.2648.
3. World Health Organization. WHO director-general's opening remarks at the media briefing on COVID-19 - 3 March 2020 [Internet]. World Health Organization; 2020 [accessed on 6 March 2020]. https://www.who.int/dg/speeches/detail/who-director-general-s-opening-remarks-at-the-media-briefing-on-covid-19---3-march-202.
4. Cavanna L, Citterio C, Toscani I, et al. Cancer patients with COVID- 19: A retrospective study of 51 patients in the district of Piacenza, Northern Italy. *Future Sci OA* 2020;24:645. doi:10.2144/fsoa-2020-0157.
5. El Saghir NS. Oncology care and education during the coronavirus (COVID-19) pandemic. AsCO Connection. 19 March 2020.
6. Liang W, Guan W, Chen R, et al. Cancer patients in SARS-CoV-2 infection: A nationwide analysis in China. *Lancet Oncol* 2020;21:335–337. doi:10.1016/S1470-2045(20)30096-6.
7. EMA. Guidance on the management of clinical trials during the COVID-19 (coronavirus) pandemic. European Medicines Agency, 2020: V3 (28/04/2020) https://health.ec.europa.eu/system/files/2022-02/guidanceclinicaltrials_covid19_en_1.pdf. Accessed 25 April 2020.
8. European Society for Medical Oncology: Cancer patient management during the COVID-19 pandemic. 2020. https://www.esmo.org/guidelines/cancer-patient-management-during-the-covid-19-pandemic.
9. Indini A, Aschele C, Cavanna L, et al. Reorganisation of medical oncology departments during the novel coronavirus disease-19 pandemic: A nationwide Italian survey. *Eur J Cancer* 2020;132:17–23. doi: 10.1016/j.ejca.2020.03.024.
10. Brandes AA, Ardizzoni A, Artioli F, et al. Fighting cancer in coronavirus disease era: Organization of work in medical oncology departments in Emilia Romagna region of Italy. *Future Oncol* 2020;16:1433–1439. doi: 10.2217/fon2020-0358.
11. Mostafaei A, Sadeghi-Ghyassi F, Kabiri N, et al. Experiences of patients and providers while using telemedicine in cancer care during COVID-19 pandemic: A systematic review and meta-synthesis of qualitative literature. *Support Care Cancer* 2022;30:10483–10494.
12. Novara G, Checcucci E, Crestani A, et al. Telehealth in urology: A systematic review of literature. How much can telemedicine be useful during and after the COVID-19 pandemic? *Eur Urol* 2020;78:786–811.
13. Hasson SP, Waissengrin B, Shachar E, et al. Rapid implementation of telemedicine during the COVID-19 pandemic: Perspectives and preferences of patients with cancer. *Oncologist* 2021;26:e679–e685.
14. Salehi F, Mashhadi L, Khazeni K, et al. Management of cancer patients in the COVID-19 crisis using telemedicine: A systematic review. *Stud Health Technol Inform* 2021;3(299):118–125. (2022). doi: 10.3233/SHTI220969.
15. Huret L, Stoekle HC, Benmaziane A, et al. Cancer and COVID-19: Ethical issues concerning the use of telemedicine during the pandemic. *BMC Health Serv Res* 2021;22:703. https://doi.org/10.1186/s12913-022-08097-w.

16. Luo J, Tong L, Crotty BH, et al. Telemedicine adoption during the COVID-19 pandemic: Gaps and inequalities. *Appl Clin Inform* 2021;12:836–844.
17. West H, Barzi A, Wong D. Telemedicine in cancer care beyond the COVID-19 pandemic: Oncology 2.0? *Curr Oncol Rep* 2022;24:1843–1850.
18. Garavand A, Aslani N, Behmanesh A, et al. Telemedicine in lung cancer during COVID-19 outbreak: A scoping review. *Am J Health Promot* 2022;11:348.

4

Estimating the COVID-19 Impact on Cancer Burden and Care in Slovenia: A Case Study

Vesna Zadnik, Sonja Tomšič, Nika Bric, Katarina Lokar, Ana Mihor, and Tina Žagar

COVID-19 Epidemic in Slovenia

A short summary of the COVID-19 epidemic in Slovenia, a middle European country with a universal health-care system, is prepared with reference to the most relevant national informers [1–5]. The measures concerning the provision of health system services were firstly enacted through the *Ordinance on temporary measures in health care to contain and control the COVID-19 epidemic* from the 20th of March 2020, which stipulated that all non-essential ambulatory visits (those not referred as needing urgent or very fast management) and elective surgery appointments are put on hold. Oncological services were listed as an exception, though all preventive care was also put on hold via the ordinance, meaning all three cancer screening programmes (cervical, breast and colorectal cancer) were temporarily stopped. In the second half of April 2020, the government began to ease restrictions (including reopening the cancer screening programmes), the restrictions on health services were lifted on 9 May 2020, and the end of the epidemic was declared on 31 May 2020. Still, some sensible measures were kept in place. Due to the rapid spread of disease among the population in autumn, an epidemic was again declared on 19 October 2020. Various measures to restrict movement, gatherings, and the provision of services have been reintroduced. In health care, all non-essential services, with the exception of oncology services, were again suspended. This time, cancer screening programmes were also part of the exception and continued to run undisturbed with some adjustments and minor changes in scope (particularly due to the lack of staff getting ill or redeployment to other wards and sites). At the end of 2020, the global development of science and services provided us with rapid antigen tests for SARS-CoV-2, which allowed for much quicker (albeit slightly less reliable) results. On 27 December 2020, the first inhabitants of Slovenia received their COVID-19 vaccine shots. In the coming months, the vaccination of the population was promoted according to the Vaccination Strategies, which defined the priority groups in line with the availability of the vaccine and other factors. The Slovenian government adjusted the measures as the epidemic progressed. The second wave of the epidemic had three peaks: the end of October 2020, the beginning

DOI: 10.1201/9781003362562-5

of January 2021, and the beginning of April 2021. On 15 June 2021, the end of epidemic was declared. Nevertheless, some measures limiting the spread of infection have remained in place. On 15 September 2021, due to the growing number of positive COVID-19 cases (pre-dominantly the Delta variant), the RVT (recovered/vaccinated/tested) rule was implemented for most services. Emergency visits and grocery stores outside shopping centres were exceptions. Alongside the RVT implementation, demand for vaccination among the general population grew. The Delta wave caused a new surge in the number of people who needed hospital treatment, especially in intensive care units (most notably during November and December 2021).

Monitoring of Cancer Burden and Care in Slovenia

Population-based cancer registries are public health entities that are established on a national or regional level for continuous systematic collection of data on the occurrence, characteristics, and outcome of reportable cancers [6]. Profound changes of cancer burden on a population level are usually observed after introducing/changing cancer screening programmes, intensive primary prevention activities addressing cancer risk factors, or significant changes in health policies, most of which we can expect and prepare for in advance to a certain degree. On rare occasions we have an opportunity to observe rapid changes in cancer burden indicators during crisis situations, for example due to catastrophes resulting in an increased exposure to certain cancer risk factors or major and/or prolonged disruptions of a country's health system, such as occur during wars or widespread epidemics.

Slovenia has a long tradition of cancer registration with the national Slovenian Cancer Registry (SCR) operating continuously since 1950. The SCR's data are important for planning and evaluation of the National Cancer Control Programme for the primary and secondary prevention of cancer, diagnostics, treatment, and rehabilitation, as well as for planning the facilities and resources needed for cancer management (staff, medical equipment, hospital facilities). The use of SCR's data is also acknowledged in Slovenian and international clinical and epidemiological research and for evaluating the effectiveness of screening programmes. In addition, more precise data on diagnosis and treatment that the SCR manages in its clinical registries can be used to monitor the quality of treatment received by cancer patients [7].

The oncological health-care system in Slovenia is highly centralised. The Institute of Oncology Ljubljana (IOL) is the only national comprehensive health centre for cancer, providing more than 80% of all systemic treatments, more than 60% of all cancer surgeries, and almost all radiotherapy treatments in Slovenia. The Hospital-Based Cancer Registry of the IOL collects data on all new patients that are admitted to the IOL for cancer diagnostics and treatment. These data are the source of valuable information for medical work and research at the IOL; at the same time, the data are promptly forwarded also to the population-based SCR, thus upgrading the central database. The University Medical Centre (UMC) Maribor is Slovenia's second oncological centre. Since 2019, the UMC Maribor has provided up-to-date information to the SCR on newly diagnosed and treated cancer patients through an online-based registration process [8]. Slovenia has a gate-keeping system in place, where the provision of secondary and tertiary health care is only possible with referrals from general practitioners. Thus, the number of referrals is an accurate reflection of demand for specialist oncological care. The e-referral system was introduced in 2017 and is maintained by the National Institute of Public Health (NIPH) [9].

Shortly after the start of the COVID-19 pandemic, an initial analysis of its impact on cancer diagnosis and care in Slovenia was published [10] using the preliminary data from the SCR and other available heath databases. To establish continuous monitoring of the effect of the COVID-19 epidemic on oncology services and cancer burden, in 2021 a web page named onKOvid (available at http://www.slora.si/en/onkovid) was launched where up-to-date indicators on cancer burden and management are available to the professional and lay public [11]. Only recently has the last follow-up study of the impact of the COVID-19 epidemic on cancer burden and care in Slovenia become available [12].

In the subsequent sections we summarise the most important conclusion from the existing publications on COVID-19's impact on cancer burden and care in Slovenia. We are providing the cancer burden and cancer care indicators for the years 2021 and 2020 in contrast to the pre-epidemic year 2019.

Cancer Burden Indicators

For the evaluation of possible delays in cancer diagnoses and the analysis of the impact of the COVID-19 epidemic on cancer burden in Slovenia, data on new cancer notifications that were provided to SCR from two major cancer centres in Ljubljana and Maribor were used. Notification of cancer has been compulsory in Slovenia since 1950; information to the SCR is provided by all Slovenian public health-care institutions, where diagnostics, treatment, and follow-up of patients are carried out. Traditionally, hospitals reported cases to the cancer registry via a special paper-based Cancer Notification Form. In 2018, the gradual transition from passive (paper) to active (web) registration allowed for up-to-date online access to cancer records in health institutions. Cancer notifications collected in the process of active registration were for the entire COVID-19 epidemic period, available to the SCR for the two main cancer centres only. The existing evaluations considered all cancers combined as well as separately the colorectal, breast, lung, prostate, non-melanoma skin cancers, skin melanoma, and lymphoma. For patients admitted to the IOL for diagnostics and/or treatment, in addition to the location of cancer, data was available also on the stage at diagnosis and the reason for the first admission at the IOL. Unlike the national cancer registry, the Hospital-Based Cancer Registry of the IOL has shorter delays in cancer registration, which allows for more detailed real-time analysis. Thus, for the cohort of patients first admitted to the IOL in 2020 and 2021, stratification was possible by gender, age group according to the age at first admission to the IOL, stage at diagnosis, and the reason for the first admission to the IOL.

There was a drop in newly diagnosed cancers in both epidemic years (2020 and 2021) in comparison to the year 2019 for most cancer sites except lung cancer (Table 4.1).

The overall number of notifications for new cancer diagnoses in the years 2020 and 2021 was lower than in 2019 for 6% and 3%, respectively. It is important to emphasise that the average growth of new cancer cases (crude incidence rate on the population level) was 2% per year before the epidemic in 2010–2019. The most prominent drops in cancer notifications were for prostate (around 20% in all years) and breast cancer (up to 25%), while notifications for lung cancer increased by over 10%.

TABLE 4.1

Change in the Number of Newly Notified Cases of Different Types of
Cancers in Years 2020 and 2021 Compared to the Pre-COVID-19 Year 2019

Cancer site	2020	2021
Colorectal	0.1 (−5.7; 6.2)	−5.0 (−10.6; 1.0)
Breast	−16.5 (−20.0; −13.0)	−12.1 (−15.7; −8.5)
Lung	13.6 (8.0; 19.5)	10.2 (4.6; 15.9)
Prostate	−21.1 (−26.0; −16.0)	−19.3 (−24.2; −14.1)
Skin, non-melanoma	−9.0 (−14.0; −3.9)	−11.2 (−16.1; −6.2)
Skin melanoma	−10.7 (−17.3; −3.7)	0.3 (−6.8; 7.7)
Stomach	−10.2 (−19.1; −0.6)	13.3 (3.3; 24.1)
Lymphoma	−6.3 (−13.3; 1.1)	−0.7 (−7.9; 6.9)
All	−6.2 (−7.7; −4.6)	−3.0 (−4.6; −1.5)

In general, drops in the monthly number of cancer notifications were more coincidental with imposed restrictions, which were more pronounced at the beginning of the observed period, than with observed surges in COVID-19 cases (Figure 4.1). The largest drop was observed in April 2020 (around 30%). The results show that the second and third wave of COVID-19 (autumn 2020, winter and spring 2021) had a smaller negative effect on the number of new cancer cases, around 10%. In the second half of 2021, the number of cancer notifications was roughly the same as in 2019. Looking at the whole period, no compensatory surges in cancer notifications are visible that would make up for the significant drops in the first, second, or third wave.

For patients admitted to the IOL for diagnostics and/or treatment, the drop was similar in males and females. The largest drop was seen in the 50–64 age group (around 15%), while for patients older than 80 years, the numbers were above expected (on average 6%).

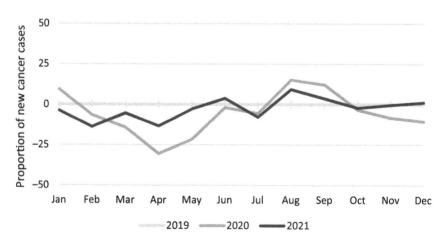

FIGURE 4.1 Proportion of new cancer cases treated in two major Slovenian hospitals in 2020 and 2021 compared to 2019.

Cancer Care Indicators

As Slovenia has a gate-keeping system in place, where secondary and tertiary care is only possible through referrals, the number of referrals is an accurate reflection of demand for specialist oncological care. The analyses of referrals for oncological examination are based on the national e-referral system, operated by NIPH. The absolute number of all monthly referrals issued in Slovenia are available for selected types of oncological health services as coded in the Codebook of Healthcare Services, namely the oncological examination – first,control, and oncological genetic testing and counselling.

In 2020, there was a drop in referrals in Slovenia for first and control oncological examination as well as for oncological genetic testing and counselling (2%, 3% and 12% respectively). Monthly fluctuations of investigated indicators are presented in Figure 4.2. The drops were first observed during the first wave (spring 2020). From June to August 2020, there was an increase in the number of control oncology examinations, but the increase did not make up for the drop in the previous months. In 2021,

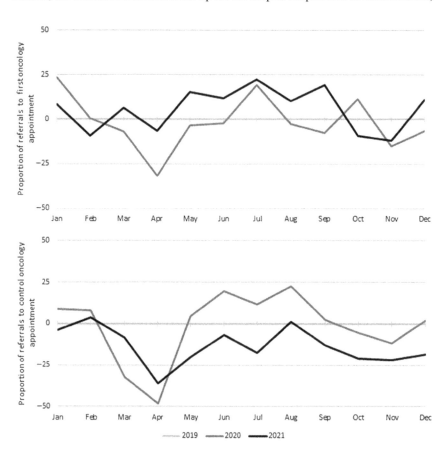

FIGURE 4.2 Proportion of referrals to first (above) and control (below) oncology appointment in Slovenia in 2020 and 2021 compared to 2019.

there was a 5.4% increase in the number of referrals for first examinations, while the number of referrals for control examinations was still significantly lower than in 2019 (-14.3%).

The analysis of the administrative data of the IOL on monthly outpatient visits, stratified according to first and control visits by divisions (medical oncology, surgery, radiotherapy), and data on cancer diagnostic imaging, namely the monthly number of X-rays, mammograms, ultrasounds, CT, MRI, and PET-CT scans performed is also available. In general, first and control outpatient visits and cancer diagnostic imaging at the IOL dropped after the onset of the COVID-19 epidemic in March 2020, but had returned to expected levels by 2021. Some deficits remain for control outpatient visits in surgical and radiotherapy departments. There were more CT, MRI, and PET-CT scans performed during the COVID-19 period than before.

Conclusion

During the COVID-19 pandemic, management of cancer in Slovenia was significantly affected. The delay in cancer services from the first wave of the epidemic has been eliminated, but we still see fewer than expected new cancer cases, which reflects disruptions in the pre-diagnostic phase and could have profound long-term consequences on cancer burden indicators. The results show that the effects of the COVID-19 epidemic on cancer management in Slovenia vary for different cancers as well as by the level of the patient-care pathway – it is probably a mixture of personal behavioural changes and systemic changes due to modifications in health-care organisation on account of COVID-19. To make incidence figures fully comparable with previous years on the population level, it is necessary to review all the notifications obtained by the SCR. Due to different disease trajectories of different cancer types, we expect different medium- and long-term effects, such as the population-based survival of cancer patients, which serves as a complex indicator reflecting the characteristics of patients as well as the organisation, accessibility, quality, and efficiency of the health-care system, and which could be examined in a few years' time. Long-term studies are already in progress.

REFERENCES

1. Leban E, Grašek M, Mozetič M, Učakar V. The COVID-19 epidemic in Slovenia. In: Vračko P, Kolar U, editors. *Public Health Achivements in Slovenia*. Ljubljana: National Institute of Public Health; 2021, p. 104.
2. Ivanuš U, Jerman T, Gašper Oblak U, Meglič L, Florjančič M, Strojan Fležar M, et al. The impact of the COVID-19 pandemic on organised cervical cancer screening: The first results of the Slovenian cervical screening programme and registry. *Lancet Reg Health Eur* 2021;5:100101. doi: 10.1016/j.lanepe.2021.100101.
3. Sledilnik.org. COVID-19 Situation in Slovenia. Project COVID-19 Tracker Slovenia [cited 2022 October 20]. Available from: https://covid-19.sledilnik.org/en/stats.
4. National Laboratory of Health, Environment and Food. Sledenje različicam SARS-CoV-2 [Monitoring of SARS-CoV-2 Variants – in Slovene].
5. IUS-INFO. Spremljamo covidne ukrepe [Monitoring of legislative concerning COVID – in Slovene] [cited 2022 October 20]. Available from: https://www.iusinfo.si/medijsko-sredisce/v-sredicu/259417.

6. Grosclaude P, Zadnik V. Population-based cancer registries: A data stream to help build an evidence-based cancer policy for Europe and for European countries. In: Launoy G, Zadnik V, Coleman MP editors. *Social Environment and Cancer in Europe: Towards an Evidence-Based Public Health Policy*. Springer: Cham, Switzerland, 2021.

7. Zadnik V, Primic Žakelj M, Lokar K, Jarm K, Ivanuš U, Žagar T. Cancer burden in Slovenia with the time trends analysis. *Radiol Oncol* 2017;51:47–55. doi: 10.1515/raon-2017-0008.

8. Cancer in Slovenia 2019. Ljubljana: Institute of Oncology Ljubljana, Epidemiology and Cancer Registry, Slovenian Cancer Registry; 2022.

9. Breznikar D. Nacionalno spremljanje čakalnih dob, mesečno poročilo za stanje na dan 1. 2. 2020 [National monitoring of waiting times, Monthly report on status on 01.02.2020 – in Slovene]. Ljubljana: National Institute of Public Health. Available from: https://www.nijz.si/sites/www.nijz.si/files/publikacije-datoteke/porocilo_enarocanje_1._2._2020_0.pdf.

10. Zadnik V, Mihor A, Tomšič S, Žagar T, Bric N, Lokar K, Oblak I. Impact of COVID-19 on cancer diagnosis and management in Slovenia – preliminary results. *Radiol Oncol* 2020;54(3):329–334. doi: 10.2478/raon-2020-0048.

11. Zadnik V, Žagar T, Bric N, Tomšič S, Mihor A, Lokar K, Jarm K. onKOvid. Epidemiology and Cancer Registry, Institute of Oncology Ljubljana [cited 2022 October 20]. Available from: http://www.slora.si/en/onkovid.

12. Žagar T, Tomšič S, Zadnik V, Bric N, Birk M, Vurzer B, Mihor A, Lokar K, Oblak I. Impact of the COVID-19 epidemic on cancer burden and cancer care in Slovenia: A follow-up study. *Radiol Oncol* 2022.

5

Clinical Analysis of COVID-19 Infections in Children with Cancer in a Tertiary Care Hospital in Bangladesh

Shahnoor Islam, Mehnaz Akter, Mohammed Tanvir Ahammed, Zannat Ara, S. M. Rezanur Rahman, AKM Khairul Basher, Kamrun Nahar, and AKM Amirul Morshed

Introduction

The aim of this chapter is to provide important data for management of COVID-19 infections in children with cancer to support frontline clinicians making data-driven decisions, prioritize government-decisions, and develop evidence-based guidelines by health-care societies and organizations.

In December 2019, China's seventh largest city of Wuhan in Hubei province became the center of a pneumonia outbreak of unknown cause, the image of which depicts severe acute respiratory syndrome coronavirus 2 (SARS-CoV-2), previously known as 2019nCoV, the novel virus that causes coronavirus disease 2019 (COVID-19). On 11 March, World Health Organization declared COVID-19 as a pandemic and till date has attacked almost all (215) the countries and states. As of 29 August 2020, a total of 24.9 million people were affected and 841,290 people killed worldwide [1]. Previous studies showed that children and adolescents with COVID-19 generally have milder disease when compared with those with cancer when infected, in addition, children had low mortality [2–4]. Severe disease has been reported in 1–6% of pediatric cases, even among cohorts, compared with 14% in adults [5–6]. Although children appear to do comparatively well, a small proportion still develop respiratory or multi-organ failure. Specifically, children and adolescents with cancer represent a potentially high-risk population for potential morbidity and mortality when infected by COVID- 19 or other respiratory viruses [7, 8]. For example, in the USA a pediatric cohorts study showed that the rate of influenza-related hospitalizations [8] in children with acute lymphoblastic leukemia (ALL) was high and was associated with increased mortality rate in these patients (about 1%) [2]. In this regard, it is necessary to evaluate clinical and health policy decision making, the clinical manifestations and outcomes of SARS-CoV-2 infection in this population due to global resource constraints, and current population-level treatment and vaccination prioritization efforts.

DOI: 10.1201/9781003362562-6

Though there is scarcity of data for children with cancer, a small number of national studies suggest disparities among countries with severe or critical infections (6.6–21%) of included patients and mortality (0–10%) [9–14]. Association of clinical risk factors with severity of COVID-19 disease in children with cancer are not well established [15]. Evaluation of global disparities in treatment and outcomes of COVID-19-related infections is necessary as 90% of children and adolescents with cancer live in low-income and middle-income countries [16]. Although children with cancer can develop a more serious illness during a respiratory virus infection such as COVID-19 than healthy children, there are only case reports or observational studies performed in individual countries, especially in high-income countries.

Bangladesh Perspectives

The first three known cases in Bangladesh were reported. On 8 March 2020, and the first death on 21 March 2020. On 6 May 2020, data obtained revealed that since the start of the outbreak, 306,794 individuals have been diagnosed with severe acute respiratory syndrome coronavirus 2 (SARS-CoV-2) and 4,174 deaths have been reported countrywide [1].

Epidemiology

An increasing number of children are being infected by SARS-CoV-2 in this pandemic [17]. Children are generally asymptomatic or pauci-symptomatic and their clinical course is shorter than adults. Therefore, children appear to be less susceptible to COVID-19 infection. Hypotheses based on children's vaccines cross reactivity against COVID-19 or on the paucity of angiotensin-converting enzyme-2 (ACE2) cell receptors present on the respiratory mucosa of children as protective factors have not been confirmed [18, 19]. Children are affected around 1-5% of diagnosed cases of COVID-19, and although children with cancer are considered a high-risk population, data specifically addressing the pediatric oncology population are still limited [20, 21].

In younger children, alterations of the immune system have been reported until 6–12 months following cessation of their antineoplastic treatment [22]. Current evidence indicates that it is not justified to interrupt or delay pediatric anticancer treatment; however, Cancer Research UK has recently proposed to stop recruiting patients in several cancer clinical trials because clinical staff are being redeployed to frontline COVID-19 care [23].

Perioperative SARS-CoV-2 infection was previously shown to be associated with significantly increased risks of morbidity and mortality. Data in the early phases of the pandemic demonstrated that peri-operative SARS-CoV-2 infection was associated with clinically important increases in mortality, in some cases more than a 10-fold increase. Notably, increased peri-operative risk remained consistently elevated until 7 weeks after SARS-CoV-2 infection, at which point it returned to baseline. Therefore, recommendations were made to delay elective surgery for 7 weeks after SARS-CoV-2 infection, unless the risks of deferring surgery outweighed the risk of postoperative morbidity or mortality associated with SARS-CoV-2 infection.

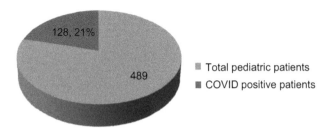

FIGURE 5.1a Number of COVID-19-positive pediatric patients among total pediatric patients. (from ref. 1 with permission)

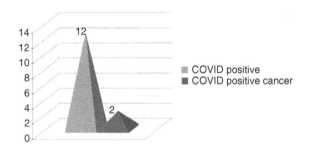

FIGURE 5.1b Number of COVID-19-positive children with cancer among COVID-19 positive pediatric patients. (from ref. 1 with permission)

As the COVID-19 pandemic has progressed, disease therapy and prevention have developed, including vaccination [24]. Variants have emerged that differ in terms of their transmissibility, the severity of illness they cause, and their ability to infect vaccinated patients.

In our study [1] a total of 24 COVID-19–positive child patients (0–12 years) with cancer were enrolled. All the admitted patients were treated COVID-19–positive. The total number of pediatric patients in the month of May, 2020 to June, 2020, were 489, among them 128 (21%) pediatric patients who were COVID positive (Figure 5.1a).

Out of 128 COVID-19-positive patients, COVID-positive pediatric cancer patients were 24 (18.75%) (Figure 5.1b).

Distribution of Disease Patterns

In our study, [1] the distribution of disease pattern with COVID-19–positive pediatric cancer patients showed that 12 (50%) patients were ALL, 4 (17%) patients were Wilms tumour, 2 (13%) patients were AML, and 1 (4%) patient was neuroblastoma, osteosarcoma, brain tumour, hepatoblastoma, and other malignancies (Figure 5.2). In the Madrid study, 11 (73%) patients were hematological cancer and 46% were acute lymphoblastic leukemia. This disease distribution is similar to our study [25].

Total number of patients 24

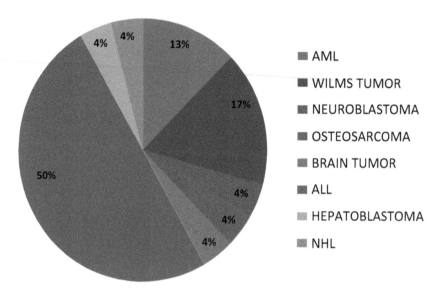

FIGURE 5.2 Disease pattern with percentages of children with cancer with COVID-19 infection. (from ref. 1 with permission)

Disease Severity

According to Sennah Mukkadah et al, [2] disease severity is classified as follows:

Critical is indicated as evidence of organ dysfunction, intubation, or death due to COVID-19.

Severe is indicated as requirement for a higher level of care for any reason or any oxygen support needed greater than regular nasal cannula or facemask, but less than intubation.

Moderate is indicated as upper respiratory tract illness requiring nasal cannula or face mask, lower respiratory tract infection with support no greater than conventional nasal cannula or facemask, no need for higher support levels for any organ system, or no need for higher level of care.

Mild is indicated as respiratory disease limited to upper respiratory tract illness on room air, any symptoms without need for higher support levels for any organ system, or no need for higher level of care.

Asymptomatic is indicated as positive test for SARS-CoV-2, and no symptoms of a respiratory or non-respiratory nature.

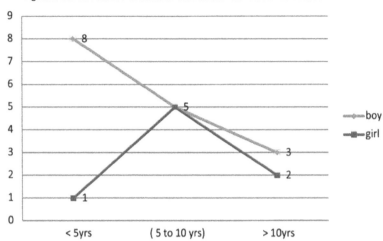

FIGURE 5.3a   Age and sex distribution of COVID-positive children with cancer. (from ref. 1 with permission)

Diagnosis

Age and Sex

For Bradley Gampel Alexandre G et al [26] shown the mean age of COVID-19 patients was 10.2 years (range 5 months to 20 years) and Elena Cela et al's study's mean age was 10.6 years (range 0–18 years). In our study, [1] 10 (42%) were in the age group 5–10 years, followed by 9 (38%) in the age group of less than 5 years and the range was from 1 to 12 years (Figure 5.3a).

Furthermore, sex distribution of COVID-19–positive children with cancer showed that a trend toward higher COVID-19-positive infection was observed in males with 16 (67%) (Figure 5.3b) than females with 8 (33%) (Figure 5.3b). Our results were similar to those of Bradley Gampel Alexandre G et al, [26] where males appeared three times more likely to have positive test results compared with females. In the Madrid study, [24] 1 out 15 was a girl. In both studies the underlying mechanism of sex discrepancy is not understood.

Symptoms and Signs

The distribution of clinical parameters among the study population showed that 11 (45%) patients presented with fever, 8 (33%) presented with running nose and cough, 5 (21%) patients had difficulty in breathing, 1 (1%) patients had diarrhoea and body ache, and 6 (25%) patients were asymptomatic (Table 5.1).

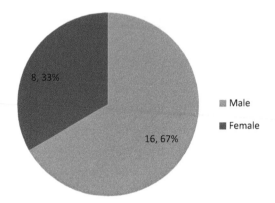

FIGURE 5.3b   Sex distribution of COVID-19 infections in children with cancer. (from ref. 1 with permission)

TABLE 5.1

Clinical Characteristics of COVID-19 in Children with Cancer

Symptoms and signs	Total (*n* = 24)	Percentage (%)
Fever	11	45
Running nose	8	33
Cough	8	33
Difficulty in breathing	5	21
Diarrhea	1	4
Bodyache	1	4
Asymptomatic		25

Source: From ref. 1 with permission.

Hematological, Biochemical Parameter, and Radiological Findings

Of the 24 cases, 17 (71%) had normal white blood cell counts, while only 2 (8%) had leukocytosis and 5 (21%) cases had leukopenia. Neutrophil counts were normal in 16 (67%) cases, neutropenia in 7 (29%) cases. Lymphocyte counts were normal in 12 (50%) cases, lymphocytosis in 2 (8%) cases, lymphocytopenia in 10 (42%) cases. C-reactive protein (CRP) was raised in 19 (79%) cases and, serum ferritin was raised in 19 (79%) cases. D-Dimer, PT and APTT were raised in 8 (33%) cases. Chest x-ray was normal in 18 (75%) cases and, abnormal in 6 (25%) cases. All the children's liver function tests and renal function tests were normal (Table 5.2).

Management of Cancer Patients

Prevention of Perioperative SARS-CoV-2 Infection: Vaccination

Vaccination is the most effective intervention and should be strongly encouraged pre-operatively to reduce the severity of infection and peri-operative complications.

TABLE 5.2

Hematological, Laboratory, Radiological Features of COVID-19 Positive Children with Cancer

Parameters	Total $N = 24$	Percentage (%)
White blood cell count, ×10⁹/L		
Increased (>10)	2	8
Normal (4–10)	17	71
Decreased (<4)	5	21
Neutrophil count, ×10⁹/L		
Increased	1	4
Normal	16	67
Decreased	7	29
Lymphocyte count, ×10⁹/L		
Increased	2	8
Normal	12	50
Decreased	10	42
C-reactive protein (1–11 mg/L)		
Normal	5	21
Raised	19	79
Serum Ferritin		
Normal	5	21
Increased	19	79
D-Dimer		
Normal	16	67
Raised	8	33
Prothrombin time		
Increased	8	33
Normal	16	67
Activated partial thromboplastin time (APTT)		
Increased	8	33
Normal	16	67
Chest x-ray		
Normal	18	75
Abnormal	6	25

Source: From ref. 1 with permission.

Vaccination with two doses has a moderate impact on reducing the severity of COVID-19, while a third vaccination dose significantly reduces the risk of infection and severity of illness [14]. Vaccination is likely to have clinical efficacy within 2 weeks and therefore patients who are partially vaccinated are likely to benefit from a further dose or doses in the pre-operative period, ideally arranged in primary care at the point of referral for consideration of surgery. If not done by the time patients have presented for surgical assessment, then vaccination should be strongly encouraged by surgical teams at this time.

Mandatory vaccination of health-care staff is currently under review as a condition of retaining or gaining such employment in the UK. Irrespective of national policy, wherever possible staff caring for patients having surgery, and particularly those who are high risk, should be vaccinated against COVID-19 [8]. Further actions to reduce the risk of SARS-CoV-2 infection include:

- Adherence by patients awaiting surgery and staff to practices that reduce the risk of community-acquired SARS-CoV-2 infection, such as mask-wearing, social distancing, hand hygiene, appropriate self-isolation and adherence to shielding advice, where indicated.
- Screening of hospital staff to prevent contact with infectious staff [9].
- Maintaining dedicated pathways that separate patients who have been screened and tested negative for SARS-CoV-2 infection from contact with patients with suspected or confirmed infection and the staff and locations involved in their treatment [10].
- Institutional implementation of environmental ventilation, air filtering, decontamination, and provision of appropriate respiratory protective equipment consistent with best practice;
- Minimising time spent by patients within health-care environments;
- Maintaining SARS-CoV-2 risk-reducing measures once discharged from hospital to avoid potential infection during the early postoperative recovery phase, which could negatively affect patient outcomes.

Treatment

In our study[1] (Table 5.3), treatment of the study population with drugs and supportive measures showed that 8 (33%) patients were treated with oral azithromycin, 16 (66%) with intravenous antibiotics, 3 (21%) with ivermectin, 4 (17%) with corticosteroid, 24 (100%) with zinc and vitamin C, 15 (63%) with blood and blood products, and (21%) patients with oxygen support. In the Madrid study none received ivermectin; instead they used hydroxychloroquine (73%), different combinations of azithromycin, corticosteroid, and remdesivir (20%), and 29 % got no treatment. Only 20% patients received oxygen support. Use of hydroxychloroquine and ivermectin is the basic difference between two studies [24].

TABLE 5.3

Drugs and Supportive Treatments with COVID-19–Positive Children with Cancer

Treatment	$N = 24$	Percentage (%)
Azithromycin	8	33
Intravenous antibiotic	16	66
Ivermectin	3	13
Corticosteroid	4	17
Oxygen support	5	21
Blood & blood product	15	63
Zinc and vitamin C	24	100

Source: From ref. 1 with permission.

Timing of Surgery after SARS-CoV-2 Infections

Given the uncertainty of the impact of variants, symptoms, and vaccinations on perioperative outcomes, elective surgery should be avoided within 7 weeks of a diagnosis of SARS-COV-2 infection, even in asymptomatic patient. This risk may be estimated by patient factors (age, comorbidities, and functional status); SARS-COV-2 infection (timing, variant, severity of initial infection, ongoing symptoms) and surgical factors (clinical priority, risk of disease progression, complexity of surgery). Shared decision-making should be done between a multidisciplinary team and the patient.

It is likely that high-income countries, through implementing the vaccination program, will be able to reduce new SARS-CoV-2 infection rates, but these countries already have tens of millions of SARS-CoV-2 infection survivors. There is limited access to SARS-CoV-2 vaccines in most of the low- and middle-income countries until at least 2023 [25]. So, this infection in pre-operative period will remain a challenge in the near future.

Elective surgery of 49 patients was delayed due to the preoperative diagnosis of asymptomatic SARS-CoV-2 infection [27]. After confirmation of a negative SARS-CoV-2 reverse transcription polymerase chain reaction (RT-PCR) nasopharyngeal swab result, patients subsequently underwent surgery. Routine surgery was postponed for pre-operative SARS-CoV-2 infected patients supported by clinical guidelines [8–9, 28, 29]. Delaying surgery beyond 7 weeks should be considered in patients with persistent symptoms and those with moderate to severe COVID-19 (e.g. those who were hospitalised) having greater risk of mortality and morbidity. In our set up, two consecutive negative SARS-CoV-2 reverse transcription polymerase chain reaction (RT-PCR) nasopharyngeal swab results 1 week apart were required for elective surgery for SARS-CoV-2-infected children with cancer.

Elective surgery should be avoided during the period that a patient may be infectious (10 days). This includes patients who test positive for SARS-CoV-2 during pre-operative screening (incidental SARS-CoV-2). Patients who are infectious pose a risk to health-care workers, other patients, and safe pathways of care. Furthermore, incidental SARS-CoV-2 may be pre-symptomatic and may be associated with increased risk of postoperative morbidity and mortality in patients having elective surgery. When emergency surgery is required during this period, full transmission-based precautions should be undertaken.

Isolation

Pre-operative isolation ≥3 days may be associated with an increased risk of postoperative pulmonary complications [14].

Anesthetic Tests

More recent evidence indicates that in patients with recent or peri-operative SARS-CoV-2 infection, local or regional anesthetic techniques may be associated with a moderate (e.g. point estimates varying between 50 and 150%) reduction in the risk of postoperative pulmonary complications and mortality when compared with general anaesthesia [14, 30].

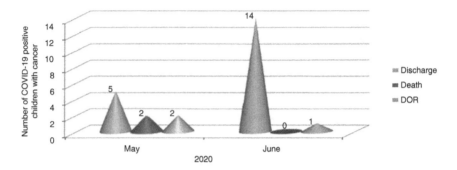

FIGURE 5.4   Outcomes of COVID-19 positive children with cancer (*y*-axis) over 2 months (*x*-axis), (from ref 1 with permission)

Outcome

There are primary (30-day postoperative mortality) and secondary outcome measures (30-day postoperative pulmonary complications). Primary outcome is a composite measure incorporating anatomical level of respiratory tract involvement (upper versus lower), respiratory support level, requirement for higher level of care for any reason, and death attributed to COVID-19. Secondary outcome is treatment modification, defined as one or more of the following: chemotherapy reduction or withheld, surgery delay, or radiotherapy delay; no changes to treatment plan or unknown treatment modification status. A Latin American survey showed interruptions in supply of blood products and chemotherapy during the pandemic, which would result in treatment modification [31].

Factors to adjust time from SARS-CoV-2 diagnosis to surgery as independent predictors of mortality in patients with peri-operative SARS-CoV-2 infection[25] included age, sex, and physical status; indication, grade, and urgency of surgery; presence of respiratory comorbidities; and national income.

In our study, [1] 19 (79%) patients were cured and discharged after receiving the COVID-19 negative reports, 3 (13%) were discharged on request, and there were 2 (8%) deaths. A total of 4 (3.8%) died who had no malignant disease (Figure 5.4).

Conclusions

Children at all ages appeared susceptible to COVID-19 and there was no significant gender difference. Although clinical manifestations of children's COVID-19 cases were generally less severe than those of adult patients. The mortality and morbidity in COVID-19 infection in children with cancer is lower than others. Surgery should be delayed for at least 7 weeks following SARS-CoV-2 infection to lessen postoperative morbidity and mortality. Patients with ongoing symptoms at ≥7 weeks from diagnosis may benefit from further delay. The impact of vaccination and new SARS-CoV-2 variants on perioperative outcomes is unclear. We recommend individualised multidisciplinary risk assessment for patients requiring elective surgery within 7 weeks of SARS-CoV-2 infection, which include baseline mortality risk calculation and assessment of risk modifiers (patient factors; SARS-CoV-2 infection; surgical factors). Two consecutive negative SARS-CoV-2 reverse transcription polymerase chain reaction (RT-PCR) nasopharyngeal swab results one week apart were required for elective surgery for SARS-CoV2-infected children with cancer in our set up. These recommendations may be updated in near future due to further study.

CONFLICT OF INTEREST
None.

CONTRIBUTORS
Funding and writing
  Shahnoor Islam and AKM Amirul Morshed

Data collection and analysis
  Shahnoor Islam, Mehnaz Akter, Mohammed Tanvir Ahammed, Zannat Ara, S. M. Rezanur Rahman, AKM Khairul Basher, Kamrun Nahar, AKM Amirul Morshed

ACKNOWLEDGMENT
We acknowledge all health-care workers involved in the diagnosis and treatment of COVID-19 patients in Bangladesh. All authors had full access to all the data in the study and had final responsibility for the decision to submit for publications.

REFERENCES
1. Islam, S., Akter, M., Ahmmed, M. T., Ara, Z., Rahman, S. R., Basher, A. K., Nahar, K., & Morshed, AKMA. Clinical analysis of COVID-19 infections in children cancer in a tertiary care hospital in Bangladesh. *J Dhaka Med Coll.* 2021;29(2):165–170. https://doi.org/10.3329/jdmc.v29i2.51193.
2. Mukkada S, Bhakta N, Chantada GL, Chen Y, Vedaraju Y, Faughnan L, Homsi MR, Muniz-Talavera H, Ranadive R, Metzger M, Friedrich P, Agulnik A, Jeha S, Lam C, Dalvi R, Hessissen L, Moreira DC, Santana VM, Sullivan M, Bouffet E, Caniza adolescents with cancer (GRCCC): A cohort study. *Lancet Oncol.* 2021 Oct;22(10):1416–1426. doi:10.1016/S1470-2045(21)00454-X.
3. Dong Y, Mo X, Hu Y, et al. Epidemiology of COVID-19 among children in China. *Pediatrics* 2020;145(6):e20200702. doi:10.1542/peds.2020-0702.
4. Mehta NS, Mytton OT, Mullins EWS, et al. SARS-CoV-2 (COVID-19): What do we know about children? A systematic review *Clin Infect Dis* 2020;71(9):2469–2479. doi:10.1093/cid/ciaa556.
5. Wu Z, McGoogan JM. Characteristics of and important lessons from the coronavirus disease 2019 (COVID-19) outbreak in China: Summary of a report of 72, 314 cases from the Chinese center for disease control and prevention. *JAMA* 2020;323(13):1239–1242. doi:10.1001/jama.2020.2648.

6. Bellino S, Punzo O, Rota MC, et al. COVID-19 disease severity risk factors for pediatric patients in Italy. *Pediatrics* 2020;146(4):e2020009399. doi:10.1542/peds.2020-009399.

7. Lee LY, Cazier JB, Angelis V, et al. COVID-19 mortality in patients with cancer on chemotherapy or other anticancer treatments: A prospective cohort study [published correction appears in Lancet. 2020 Aug 22;396(10250):534]. *Lancet* 2020;395(10241):1919–1926. doi:10.1016/S0140-6736(20)31173-9.

8. Lee GE, Fisher BT, Xiao R, Coffin SE, Feemster K, Seif AE, Bagatell R, Li Y, Huang YS, Aplenc R. Burden of influenza-related hospitalizations and attributable mortality in pediatric acute lymphoblastic leukemia. *J Pediatric Infect Dis Soc* 2015 December;4(4):290–296. doi:10.1093/jpids/piu066.

9. Bisogno G, Provenzi M, Zama D, et al. Clinical characteristics and outcome of severe acute respiratory syndrome coronavirus 2 infection in Italian pediatric oncology patients: A study from the infectious diseases working group of the Associazione Italiana di Oncologia e Ematologia Pediatric. *J Pediatric Infect Dis Soc* 2020 July 11;9:530–534. doi: 10.1093/jpids/piaa088.

10. Montoya J, Ugaz C, Alarcon S, et al. COVID-19 in pediatric cancer patients in a resource-limited setting: National data from Peru. *Pediatr Blood Cancer* 2021;68(2):e28610. doi:10.1002/pbc.28610.

11. Rouger-Gaudichon J, Thébault E, Félix A, et al. Impact of the first wave of COVID-19 on pediatric oncology and hematology: A report from the French society of pediatric oncology. *Cancers* 2020;12(11):3398. Published 2020 Nov 17. doi:10.3390/cancers12113398.

12. Kebudi R, Kurucu N, Tuğcu D, et al. COVID-19 infection in children with cancer and stem cell transplant recipients in Turkey: A nationwide study. *Pediatr Blood Cancer* 2021;68(6):e28915. doi:10.1002/pbc.28915.

13. Millen GC, Arnold R, Cazier JB, et al. Severity of COVID-19 in children with cancer: Report from the United Kingdom paediatric coronavirus cancer monitoring project. *Br J Cancer* 2021;124(4):754–759. doi:10.1038/s41416-020-01181-0.

14. André N, Rouger-Gaudichon J, Brethon B, et al. COVID-19 in pediatric oncology from French pediatric oncology and hematology centers: High risk of severe forms? *Pediatr Blood Cancer* 2020;67(7):e28392. doi:10.1002/pbc.28392.

15. Chiotos K, Hayes M, Kimberlin DW, et al. Multicenter interim guidance on use of antivirals for children with coronavirus disease 2019/severe acute respiratory syndrome coronavirus 2. *J Pediatric Infect Dis Soc* 2021;10(1):34–48. doi:10.1093/jpids/piaa115.

16. Ward ZJ, Yeh JM, Bhakta N, Frazier AL, Atun R. Estimating the total incidence of global childhood cancer: A simulation-based analysis. *Lancet Oncol* 2019;20(4):483–493. doi:10.1016/S1470-2045(18)30909-4.

17. Bai K, Liu W, Liu C, et al. Clinical analysis of 25 COVID-19 infections in children. *Pediatr Infect Dis J* 2020;39(7):e100–e103. doi:10.1097/INF.0000000000002740.

18. Yu Y, Jin H, Chen Z, et al. Children's vaccines do not induce cross reactivity against SARS-CoV. *J Clin Pathol* 2007;60(2):208–211. doi:10.1136/jcp.2006.038893.

19. Lu R, Zhao X, Li J, Niu P, Yang B, Wu H, Tan W et al. Genomic characterization and epidemiology of 2019 novel corona virus: Implications for virus origins and receptor binding. *Lancet* 2020;395(10224):P565574. doi:10.1016/S0140-6736(20)30251-8.

20. Bouffet E, Challinor J, Sullivan M, Biondi A, Rodriguez-Galindo C, Pritchard-Jones K. Early advice on managing children with cancer during the COVID.-19 pandemic and a call for sharing experiences. *Pediatr Blood Cancer* 2020;67(7):e28327. doi:10.1002/pbc.28327.

21. Ludvigsson JF. Systematic review of COVID-19 in children shows milder cases and a better prognosis than adults. *Acta Paediatr* 2020;109(6):1088–1095. doi:10.1111/apa.15270.

22. Ruggiero A, Romano A, Attina G. Facing the COVID19 outbreak in children with cancer. *Drugs in Context* 2020;9: April 12 2020. https://doi.org/10.7573/dic.2020-4-12.

23. Thornton J. Clinical trials suspended in UK to prioritize COVID-19 studies and free staff. *BMJ* 2020; 368:m1173. doi: https://doi.org/10.1136/bmj.m1172.

24. de Rojas T, Pérez-Martínez A, Cela E, Baragaño M, Galán V, Mata C, Peretó A, Madero L. COVID-19 infection in children and adolescents with cancer in Madrid. *Pediatric Blood Cancer* 2020; 67(7) e28397 https:/doi.org/10.1002/pbc.28397.

25. COVIDSurg Collaborative and GlobalSurg Collaborative. *Timing of surgery following SARS-CoV-2* infection: An international prospective cohort study. *Anesthesia* 2020; 76(6):748–758. doi: 10.1111/anae.15458.

26. Bradley GAG et al. (2020). COVID-19 disease in New York city pediatric hematology and oncology patients. *Pediatr Blood Cancer* 2020;67(9): https://doi.org/10.1002/pbc.284.

27. Liang W, Guan W, Chen R, et al. Cancer patients in SARS-CoV-2 infection: A nationwide analysis in China. *Lancet Oncol* 2020;21(3):335–337. doi:10.1016/S1470-2045(20)30096-6.

28. Saini KS, Tagliamento M, Lambertini M, et al. Mortality in patients with cancer and coronavirus disease 2019: A systematic review and pooled analysis of 52 studies. *Eur J Cancer* 2020;139:43–50. doi:10.1016/j.ejca.2020.08.011.

29. Rüthrich MM, Giessen-Jung C, Borgmann S, et al. COVID-19 in cancer patients: Clinical characteristics and outcome-an analysis of the LEOSS registry. *Ann Hematol* 2021;100(2):383–393. doi:10.1007/s00277-020-04328-4.

30. Moreira DC, Sniderman E, Mukkada S, et al. The global COVID-19 observatory and resource center for childhood cancer: A response for the pediatric oncology community by SIOP and St. Jude Global. *Pediatr Blood Cancer* 2021;68(5):e28962. doi:10.1002/pbc.28962.

31. Vasquez L, Sampor C, Villanueva G, et al. Early impact of the COVID-19 pandemic on paediatric cancer care in Latin America. *Lancet Oncol* 2020;21(6):753–755. doi:10.1016/S1470-2045(20)30280-1.

6

The Relationship between Lung Cancer and SARS-CoV-2 Infection

Abhishek Shankar, Deepak Saini, Abhijit Chakraborty, Sachidanand Jee Bharati, Chandra Prakash Prasad, Mayank Singh, Pritanjali Singh, Amrita Rakesh, Rohit Saini, and Rakesh Ranjan

Introduction

As per GLOBOCAN 2020, with over 2.3 million new cases comprising about 11% of total cancer incidence and nearly 1.8 million deaths accounting for 18% of total cancer related, lung cancer stands on top in cancer-related mortality worldwide [1]. Advancements in treatment and screening methods for lung cancer have led to an increase in the number of lung cancer patient survivors, though overall survival remains poor in comparison to other cancers. Recurrence in cases of lung cancer is an important issue, thus routine follow-up and screening are needed [2–4]. Since early 2020, the coronavirus (COVID-19) pandemic caused by severe acute respiratory syndrome coronavirus 2 (SARS-CoV-2) has affected all aspects of healthcare delivery, and diagnostics and treatment for lung cancer have become more complex and present unique challenges. There had been a significant reduction in patients being assessed for cancers in general and lung cancer in particular during the pandemic, partially due to lockdowns and poor access to healthcare facilities for non-COVID patients. The advanced stage of presentation with vulnerability to catching infection presented a challenge for lung cancer management during COVID-19, along with the more severe presentation of COVID-19 in lung cancer patients. Many of the symptoms are commonly presented in cases of both lung cancer and coronavirus infection, making it clinically challenging to diagnose the correct disease [5–8]. The mortality rate was reported three times higher among cancer patients in comparison to patients without cancer [9]. In lung cancer patients, pathological changes in lung tissues increase the chances of acquiring the infection. This can explain the increased severity of COVID-19 in lung cancer patients leading to higher mortality among lung cancer patients [5].

Risk of COVID-19 in Cancer Patients

Many pieces of literature reported increased hospitalisation and higher severity of COVID-19 in patients with cancer, particularly lung cancer [5–7]. A longer course of recovery and severity of COVID-19 among lung cancer patients was reported. Only

DOI: 10.1201/9781003362562-7

about 30% of lung cancer patients were found with mild COVID-19 infection while over 65% had severe SARS-CoV-2 infection and were hospitalised. Mortality in lung cancer patients due to COVID-19 was reported at around 25%. Less smoking habits (fewer packs per year) and no history of obstructive pulmonary diseases were factors reported in lung cancer patients having COVID-19 who recovered. There was a challenge to differentiate between similar lesions found in lung cancer and COVID-19.

Studies from China, where the first outbreak was reported, found severe infection in patients with lung cancer. Advanced-stage of lung cancer and older age were associated with unfavorable outcomes. In the area of the first outbreak, nearly one-fifth of patients who needed hospitalisation had lung cancer and these patients accounted for around 18% of mortality due to COVID-19. The severity of SARS-CoV-2 infection, higher rate of ICU admission, and use of mechanical ventilation were also reported among lung cancer patients [7, 10–12]. Long-term residual symptoms of COVID-19 were reported in patients with a lower diffusing capacity of the lung for carbon monoxide (DLCO) [13]. Also, DLCO is reported to be associated with lung cancer [14]. Meta-analysis studies reported a higher rate of mortality among lung cancer patients than other cancer types. These meta-analyses have found significantly higher mortality among lung cancer patients with COVID-19 than patients having only COVID-19. However, the mortality rate was not significantly different in comparison with COVID-19 patients having haematological cancer. In this study, of all the COVID-19 cases, a little over 2% of cases had lung cancer and pre- and post-COVID-19 outbreak, and no significant increase in advanced-stage lung cancer cases was reported [5, 15].

How Do the Symptoms of COVID-19 and Lung Cancer Compare?

Lung cancer and COVID-19 share many symptoms. However, each condition also has unique symptoms as well. Table 6.1 can help give you an idea of which symptoms are common and which are unique.

Lung Cancer and COVID-19 Mechanism

In lung cancer, inflammation plays an important role in the development of malignancy by immunosuppression, creating a microenvironment for malignancy and metastasis. Chronic unregulated inflammation creates a tumour microenvironment (TME) which is closely related to the development of carcinogenesis. Inflammation produces factors such as Interleukin (IL-1) and TNF-α, which damage the alveolar lining [16–18]. In SARS-CoV-2 infection, changes are found in alveolar epithelium, type-II pneumocytes, and hyaline membranes. Thickening of alveolar lining, formation of hyaline membrane, exudate, and damage to epithelium with hyperplasia of pneumocytes was reported. Expression of Angiotensin-converting enzyme 2 (ACE-2) is found elevated in lung cancer patients, which is associated with a history of smoking and aging. In the advanced stage of presentation, pneumonia, and consolidation were also reported. Studies indicated binding SARS-CoV-2 to ACE2 receptors for replication [7, 19]. In lung cancer, an already weak and susceptible cellular environment offers an opportunity for infection such as COVID-19 to further damage the cells, leading the higher severity [16].

TABLE 6.1

Differential Listing of Symptoms

	Lung cancer	COVID-19
Cough	✓	✓
Shortness of breath	✓	✓
Fatigue	✓	✓
Chest pain	✓	✓ (severe cases)
Wheezing	✓	
Hoarseness	✓	
Coughing up blood	✓	
Reduced appetite	✓	
Unintentional weight loss	✓	
Recurrent or persistent lung infections	✓	
Fever, with or without chills		✓
Muscle pain		✓
Headache		✓
Runny or stuffy nose		✓
Sore throat		✓
Loss of smell and taste		✓
Nausea or vomiting		✓
Diarrhoea		✓

Smoking, Lung Cancer, and COVID-19

Smoking is a major risk factor for lung cancer incidence and around 80–90% of cases of lung cancer can directly be attributed to smoking. There are 30 times increased risk of cancer development in smokers in comparison to non-smokers. Reactive oxygen species (ROS) and carcinogens presented in smoking damage the tissue lining of the lungs leading to inflammation [20]. Smoking is also a risk factor in cases of influenza and the risk is five times higher than non-smokers. Cases and severity of COVID-19 was reported much higher in patients with a history of smoking than in non-smokers, who have a relative risk of 2.4 [21]. A study reported higher recovery in lung cancer patients with less habit of smoking history [6].

Smoking is inversely associated with DLCO. Lower levels of DLCO were found to be associated with a longer duration of COVID-19 among adults [13, 14]. Smoking plays an important role in the pathogenesis of inflammation in lung cancer. These changes cause the release of many factors such as interleukin (IL), prostaglandin (PG), cytokines, and transforming growth factor (TGF), leading to cell injury [20]. Higher hospital admission was reported in patients with COVID-19 having a history of tobacco smoking. Studies reported that ACE-2 gene expression also increases the susceptibility to catching COVID-19 through droplet infection. Higher severity of COVID-19 was reported in patients with lung cancer [5, 7].

Diagnostic Challenge: Lung Cancer and COVID-19

SARS-CoV-2 infection posed a challenge to oncologists in the diagnosis of lung cancer. In patients presenting with symptoms of fever, cough, fatigue, and dyspnoea, oncologists found difficulties in differentiating between lung cancer and COVID-19. Invasive techniques for lung cancer diagnosis had major restrictions during the COVID-19 outbreak to control the infection. Another challenge was to differentiate between drug-induced pneumonia and pneumonia due to COVID-19 infection. Asymptomatic patients were accidentally diagnosed with COVID-19 during routine diagnostic examinations for cancer. There was a challenge to differentiate similar lesions found in lung cancer and COVID-19 patients such as single and multiple pure ground-glass lesions, crazy paving opacities, consolidations, and pneumonia [7, 22–25].

Dilemma with Reporting Lung Metastasis

There are difficulties in reporting lung metastasis in cancer patients who present with a sub-centimetre lesion on the chest CT with a history of COVID-19 infection in the post-pandemic era. Lung cancer patients with newly developed bilateral multiple ground-glass opacities with consolidations predominantly present in the peripheral lung are difficult to report as it may be either COVID-19 pneumonia or tumour progression. Abnormal chest shadows seen in patients receiving immune checkpoint inhibitors are often difficult to diagnose because of various possible causes, such as immune-related pneumonitis, tumor progression, and tumour pseudoprogression [26]. CT findings of COVID-19 pneumonia can also overlap with those of treatment-related pneumonitis, which is seen in immunotherapy and molecular-targeted therapy [27, 28]. At present, it is impossible to exclude COVID-19 pneumonia based on radiological findings, and this is an important consideration to treat lung metastasis in the post-pandemic world.

Potential Drug that has a Symmetrical Effect on Lung Cancer and COVID-19

Bradykinin is a physiologically and pharmacologically active peptide of the kinin group of proteins, consisting of nine amino acids. It has multiple pathophysiologic functions such as induction of vascular permeability and mitogenesis, and it triggers the release of other mediators such as nitric oxide in inflammatory and cancer tissues [29]. Bradykinin-mediated signalling activates pro-inflammatory cytokines storms. These cytokines are implicated in different clinical inflammatory conditions including fibrosis, cardiovascular diseases, lung cancer, and severe acute respiratory syndrome coronavirus 2 (SARS-CoV-2) [30, 31]. Recent studies show that angiotensin-converting enzyme inhibitors (ACEIs), which are mainly used to treat high blood pressure, increase the risk of lung cancer [32]. Bradykinin antagonists have clinical potential for the treatment of human lung cancers [33]. Bradykinin is also found to trigger SARS-CoV-2 infection [34]. All of these findings suggested that as a molecule, bradykinin has immense therapeutic value. Therefore, there is a need to fill the gap and identify the bradykinin-mediated signalling mechanisms and therapeutic approach.

Recently chloroquine (CQ) has been implicated as a chemotherapeutic agent against different cancers [35–39]. A hydroxylation compound of CQ, hydroxychloroquine (HCQ) has also been reported to suppress lung cancer by promoting M1 macrophages and inducing the CD8+ T cell antitumour effect [40]. A few clinical trials [41, 42] reported that HCQ is a potential drug against non-small cell lung cancer (NSCLC). HCQ has also been demonstrated to have anti-SARS-CoV activity in vitro [43]. Researchers from China reported that chloroquine and hydroxychloroquine inhibit SARS-CoV-2 in vitro with a dose of EC50 = 5.47% μM and EC50 = 0.72% μM respectively. This data established that HCQ has more potential than CQ to treat SARS-CoV-2. A recent clinical trial [44] published results that established COVID-19 patients to be treated with HCQ and azithromycin to cure their infection and to limit the transmission of the virus to other people in order to prevent the spread [45].

Genetic diversity was identified in lung cancer, including mutations in Ki-ras2 Kirsten rat sarcoma viral oncogene homolog (KRAS), epidermal growth factor receptor (EGFR), B-RAF (BRAF), and phosphatidylinositol 3-kinase (PI3K) signalling [46]. A study reported that HIV-positive patients have a high risk of developing non-small cell lung carcinoma (NSCLC) compared to the same age group in the general population [47]. Lopinavir/ritonavir (LPV/r) are well-established drugs for HIV treatment that block the ability of HIV to make copies of itself. A few in vitro studies reported in 2020 [48, 49] that LPV/r can prevent lung cancer by enhancing apoptosis, and induction of indication of cellular stress, cytotoxicity, and DNA damage within the cell. A combination of LPV/r is one of the repurposed drugs currently used in the treatment of COVID-19 [50]. However, a clinical trial report from China [51] (Chinese Clinical Trial Register number, ChiCTR2000029308) has reported that LPV/r has no effect in hospitalised adult patients with severe COVID-19.

Tocilizumab, a humanised recombinant monoclonal interleukin 6 receptor (IL-6R) antibody is approved to treat cytokine release syndrome (CRS), which is severe or life-threatening. Stroud et al. show tocilizumab would be a promising drug for immune checkpoint blockade [52]. This drug has been well studied to treat NSCLC [53] in vitro. A phase II clinical trial is underway to investigate the effect of tocilizumab in locally advanced NSCLC [54]. In 2021, Bonomi et al. [53] presented a case report which suggests that tocilizumab can be safely used to treat COVID-19-infected patients. The RECOVERY trial recommends adding tocilizumab to dexamethasone in patients who have rapidly increased oxygen needs and systemic inflammation [55]. In the REMAP-CAP trial [56], tocilizumab has been used in combination with corticosteroids that reduce the mortality of COVID-19–infected patients who were admitted to the ICU. Both REMAP-CAP and RECOVERY evaluated the efficacy of adding tocilizumab to standard care; in both cases, standard care included dexamethasone therapy. A Phase II clinical trial [57] that included 920 patients has reported that tocilizumab reduced the lethality rate without significant toxicity in patients with COVID-19.

Remdesivir is a nucleotide analog GS-5734 that has an anti-coronal virus effect that established the in-vivo models [58]. This drug is produced by the biotechnology company Gilead. In the in vivo mice model, it has been reported that remdesivir can improve lung function by reducing the pathology and viral load [59]. A report from the United States show that a patient with COVID-19 survived after remdesivir treatment [60]. At the same time, another study reported that after the use of remdesivir, the mortality rate decreased in patients with COVID-19 [61]. However, this study has no control group that can be used to make a proper scientific conclusion. A Phase III clinical trial completed in December 2020 [62] fails to show a significant improvement in patients treated with remdesivir. However, depending on the results of another trial [63], this drug has been approved for sale to the public for the treatment of SARS-CoV-2 infection (COVID-19).

Conclusion

This chapter summarises the few similarities in mechanism, clinical and radiological presentation, disease progression, and potential drug treatment between lung cancer and COVID-19. Patients with lung cancer need regular clinical and radiologic examinations and follow-ups, which might be hampered by the COVID-19 pandemic. Radiological findings due to COVID-19 infection have put oncologists in a dilemma as it mimics disease progression and the effects of therapy.

REFERENCES

1. GLOBOCAN 2020. Available from: https://gco.iarc.fr/today.
2. Rajapakse P. An update on survivorship issues in lung cancer patients. *World J Oncol* 2021;12(2–3):45–49.
3. Sim J-A, Kim YA, Kim JH, Lee JM, Kim MS, Shim YM, et al. The major effects of health-related quality of life on 5-year survival prediction among lung cancer survivors: Applications of machine learning. *Sci Rep* 2020;10(1):10693.
4. Yang P. Epidemiology of lung cancer prognosis: Quantity and quality of life. *Methods Mol Biol* 2009;471:469–486.
5. Wang L, Wang Y, Cheng X, Li X, Li J. Impact of coronavirus disease 2019 on lung cancer patients: A meta-analysis. *Transl Oncol* 2023;28:101605.
6. Luo J, Rizvi H, Preeshagul IR, Egger JV, Hoyos D, Bandlamudi C, et al. COVID-19 in patients with lung cancer. *Ann Oncol* 2020;31(10):1386–1396.
7. Shankar A, Saini D, Bhandari R, Bharati SJ, Kumar S, Yadav G, et al. Lung cancer management challenges amidst COVID-19 pandemic: Hope lives here. *Lung Cancer Manag* 2020;9(3):LMT33.
8. Shankar A, Saini D, Goyal N, Roy S, Angural H, et al. Cancer care delivery challenges in India during the COVID-19 era: Are we prepared for the postpandemic shock? *Asia Pac J Oncol Nurs* 2021;8(1):1–4.
9. Parise R, Li YE, Nadar RM, Ramesh S, Ren J, Govindarajulu MY, et al. Health influence of SARS-CoV-2 (COVID-19) on cancer: A review *Acta Biochim Biophys Sin* 2022;54(10):1395–1405.
10. Tian J, Yuan X, Xiao J, Zhong Q, Yang C, Liu B, et al. Clinical characteristics and risk factors associated with COVID-19 disease severity in patients with cancer in Wuhan, China: A multicentre, retrospective, cohort study. *Lancet Oncol* 2020;21(7):893–903.
11. Dai M, Liu D, Liu M, Zhou F, Li G, Chen Z, et al. Patients with cancer appear more vulnerable to SARS-CoV-2: A multicenter study during the COVID-19 outbreak. *Cancer Discov* 2020;10(6):783–791.
12. Passaro A, Bestvina C, Velez Velez M, Garassino MC, Garon E, Peters S. Severity of COVID-19 in patients with lung cancer: Evidence and challenges. *J Immunother Cancer* 2021;9(3).
13. Bellan M, Apostolo D, Albè A, Crevola M, Errica N, Ratano G, et al. Determinants of long COVID among adults hospitalized for SARS-CoV-2 infection: A prospective cohort study. 2022;13.

14. Ventura L, Gnetti L, Milanese G, Rossi M, Leo L, Cattadori S, et al. Relationship between the diffusing capacity of the lung for carbon monoxide (DLCO) and lung adenocarcinoma patterns: New possible insights. *Res Sq.* 2020;(Preprinit):doi: 10.21203/rs.3.rs-1721783/v1.

15. Peravali M, Joshi I, Ahn J, Kim C. A systematic review and meta-analysis of clinical characteristics and outcomes in patients with lung cancer with coronavirus disease 2019. *JTO Clin Res Rep* 2021;2(3):100141.

16. Malkani N, Rashid MU. SARS-COV-2 infection and lung tumor microenvironment. *Mol Biol Rep* 2021;48(2):1925–1934.

17. Zhao H, Wu L, Yan G, Chen Y, Zhou M, Wu Y, et al. Inflammation and tumor progression: Signaling pathways and targeted intervention. *Signal Transduct Target Ther* 2021;6(1):263.

18. Tan Z, Xue H, Sun Y, Zhang C, Song Y, Qi Y. The role of tumor inflammatory microenvironment in lung cancer. *Front Pharmacol* 2021;12:688625.

19. Tian S, Xiong Y, Liu H, Niu L, Guo J, Liao M, et al. Pathological study of the 2019 novel coronavirus disease (COVID-19) through postmortem core biopsies. *Mod Pathol* 2020;33(6):1007–1014.

20. Walser T, Cui X, Yanagawa J, Lee JM, Heinrich E, Lee G, et al. Smoking and lung cancer: The role of inflammation. *Proc Am Thorac Soc* 2008;5(8):811–815.

21. Ackermann M, Verleden SE, Kuehnel M, Haverich A, Welte T, Laenger F, et al. Pulmonary vascular endothelialitis, thrombosis, and angiogenesis in Covid-19. *N Engl J Med* 2020;383(2):120–128.

22. Xu C, Li L, Wang W. Challenges in advanced lung cancer diagnosis during the COVID-19 pandemic. *Technol Cancer Res Treat* 2021;20:15330338211050764.

23. Catania C, Stati V, Spitaleri G. Interstitial pneumonitis in the COVID-19 era: A difficult differential diagnosis in patients with lung cancer. *Tumori* 2021;107(3):267–269.

24. Guarnera A, Santini E, Podda P. COVID-19 pneumonia and lung cancer: A challenge for the radiologist review of the main radiological features, differential diagnosis and overlapping pathologies. *Tomography* 2022;8(1):513–528.

25. Round T, L'Esperance V, Bayly J, Brain K, Dallas L, Edwards JG, et al. COVID-19 and the multidisciplinary care of patients with lung cancer: An evidence-based review and commentary. *Br J Cancer* 2021;125(5):629–640.

26. Masuhiro K, Shiroyama T, Nagatomo I, Kumanogoh A. Unique case of pseudoprogression manifesting as lung cavitation after pembrolizumab treatment. *J Thorac Oncol* 2019;14(5):e108–e109.

27. Calabrò L, Peters S, Soria JC, Di Giacomo AM, Barlesi F, Covre A, et al. Challenges in lung cancer therapy during the COVID-19 pandemic. *Lancet Respir Med* 2020;8(6):542–544.

28. Chang HL, Chen YH, Taiwan HC, Yang CJ. EGFR tyrosine kinase inhibitor-associated interstitial lung disease during the coronavirus disease 2019 pandemic. *J Thorac Oncol* 2020;15(8):e129–e131.

29. Wu J, Akaike T, Hayashida K, Miyamoto Y, Nakagawa T, Miyakawa K, et al. Identification of bradykinin receptors in clinical cancer specimens and murine tumor tissues. *Int J Cancer* 2002;98(1):29–35.

30. Couture R, Harrisson M, Vianna RM, Cloutier F. Kinin receptors in pain and inflammation. *Eur J Pharmacol* 2001;429(1–3):161–176.

31. Rex DAB, Deepak K, Vaid N, Dagamajalu S, Kandasamy RK, Flo TH, et al. A modular map of bradykinin-mediated inflammatory signaling network. *J Cell Commun Signal* 2022;16(2):301–310.

32. Hicks BM, Filion KB, Yin H, Sakr L, Udell JA, Azoulay L. Angiotensin converting enzyme inhibitors and risk of lung cancer: Population-based cohort study. *BMJ* 2018;363:k4209.

33. Stewart JM, Gera L, Chan DC, York EJ, Stewart LT, Simkeviciene V, et al. New lung cancer drugs from bradykinin antagonists. *Chest* 2004;125(5 Suppl):148s.

34. Rex DAB, Vaid N, Deepak K, Dagamajalu S, Prasad TSK. A comprehensive review on current understanding of bradykinin in COVID-19 and inflammatory diseases. *Mol Biol Rep* 2022;49(10):9915–9927.

35. Maes H, Kuchnio A, Peric A, Moens S, Nys K, De Bock K, et al. Tumor vessel normalization by chloroquine independent of autophagy. *Cancer Cell* 2014;26(2):190–206.

36. Pascolo S. Time to use a dose of chloroquine as an adjuvant to anti-cancer chemotherapies. *Eur J Pharmacol* 2016;771:139–144.

37. Sotelo J, Briceño E, López-González MA. Adding chloroquine to conventional treatment for glioblastoma multiforme: A randomized, double-blind, placebo-controlled trial. *Ann Intern Med* 2006;144(5):337–343.

38. Maastricht Radiation Oncology. Chloroquine as an Anti-Autophagy Drug in Stage IV Small Cell Lung Cancer (SCLC) Patients (Chloroquine IV): ClinicalTrials.gov Identifier: NCT00969306; Sept 2009. Available from: https://clinicaltrials.gov/ct2/show/NCT00969306.

39. Maastricht Radiation Oncology. The Addition of Chloroquine to Chemoradiation for Glioblastoma: ClinicalTrials.gov Identifier: NCT02432417; May 2015. Available from: https://clinicaltrials.gov/ct2/show/NCT02432417.

40. Li Y, Cao F, Li M, Li P, Yu Y, Xiang L, et al. Hydroxychloroquine induced lung cancer suppression by enhancing chemo-sensitization and promoting the transition of M2-TAMs to M1-like macrophages. *J Exp Clin Cancer Res* 2018;37(1):259.

41. Abramson Cancer Center of the University of Pennsylvania. Binimetinib and Hydroxychloroquine in Patients With Advanced KRAS Mutant Non-Small Cell Lung Cancer: ClinicalTrials.gov Identifier: NCT04735068; Feb 2021. Available from: https://clinicaltrials.gov/ct2/show/NCT04735068.

42. Haematology-Oncology – National University Hospital Singapore. Hydroxychloroquine and Gefitinib to Treat Lung Cancer: ClinicalTrials.gov Identifier: NCT00809237; Dec 2008. Available from: https://clinicaltrials.gov/ct2/show/NCT00809237

43. Shimizu H, Mimoto K, Yokoyama T. Topological difference in the three-dimensional sinusoid structure between normal human liver and hepatocellular carcinoma. *Microvasc Res* 1991;42(3):280–287.

44. Samuel Brown Intermountain Health Care Inc. Hydroxychloroquine vs. Azithromycin for Hospitalized Patients With Suspected or Confirmed COVID-19 (HAHPS): ClinicalTrials.gov Identifier: NCT04329832; Apr 2022. Available from: https://clinicaltrials.gov/ct2/show/NCT04329832.

45. Gautret P, Hoang VT, Lagier JC, Raoult D. Effect of hydroxychloroquine and azithromycin as a treatment of COVID-19: Results of an open-label non-randomized clinical trial, an update with an intention-to-treat analysis and clinical outcomes. *Int J Antimicrob Agents* 2021;57(1):106239.

46. Cooper WA, Lam DC, O'Toole SA, Minna JD. Molecular biology of lung cancer. *J Thorac Dis* 2013;5(Suppl 5):S479–S490.

47. Koegelenberg CF, Van der Made T, Taljaard JJ, Irusen EM. The impact of HIV infection on the presentation of lung cancer in South Africa *S Afr Med J* 2016;106(7):666–668.

48. Marima R, Hull R, Dlamini Z, Penny C. Efavirenz and lopinavir/ritonavir alter cell cycle regulation in lung cancer. *Front Oncol* 2020;10:1693.

49. Marima R, Hull R, Dlamini Z, Penny C. The dual protease inhibitor lopinavir/ritonavir (LPV/r) exerts genotoxic stress on lung cells. *Biomed Pharmacother* 2020;132:110829.

50. Nutho B, Mahalapbutr P, Hengphasatporn K, Pattaranggoon NC, Simanon N, Shigeta Y, et al. Why are lopinavir and ritonavir effective against the newly emerged coronavirus 2019? atomistic insights into the inhibitory mechanisms. *Biochemistry* 2020;59(18):1769–1779.

51. A randomized, controlled open-label trial to evaluate the efficacy and safety of lopinavir-ritonavir in hospitalized patients with novel coronavirus pneumonia (COVID-19): Chinese Clinical Trial Register number, ChiCTR2000029308; Apr 2020. Available from: https://covid-19.cochrane.org/studies/crs-13247564.

52. Stroud CR, Hegde A, Cherry C, Naqash AR, Sharma N, Addepalli S, et al. Tocilizumab for the management of immune mediated adverse events secondary to PD-1 blockade. *J Oncol Pharm Pract* 2019;25(3):551–557.

53. Kim NH, Kim SK, Kim DS, Zhang D, Park JA, Yi H, et al. Anti-proliferative action of IL-6R-targeted antibody tocilizumab for non-small cell lung cancer cells. *Oncol Lett* 2015;9(5):2283–2288.

54. M.D. Anderson Cancer Center. Tocilizumab, Ipilimumab, and Nivolumab for the Treatment of Advanced Melanoma, Non-Small Cell Lung Cancer, or Urothelial Carcinoma: ClinicalTrials.gov Identifier: NCT04940299; June 2021. Available from: https://clinicaltrials.gov/ct2/show/NCT04940299.

55. Horby P, Lim WS, Emberson JR, Mafham M, Bell JL, Linsell L, et al. Dexamethasone in hospitalized patients with Covid-19. *N Engl J Med* 2021;384(8):693–704.

56. Gordon AC, Mouncey PR, Al-Beidh F, Rowan KM, Nichol AD, Arabi YM, et al. Interleukin-6 receptor antagonists in critically ill patients with Covid-19. *N Engl J Med* 2021;384(16):1491–1502.

57. National Cancer Institute Naples. Tocilizumab in COVID-19 Pneumonia (TOCIVID-19) (TOCIVID-19): ClinicalTrials.gov Identifier: NCT04317092; March 2020. Available from: https://clinicaltrials.gov/ct2/show/NCT04317092.

58. Warren TK, Jordan R, Lo MK, Ray AS, Mackman RL, Soloveva V, et al. Therapeutic efficacy of the small molecule GS-5734 against Ebola virus in rhesus monkeys. *Nature* 2016;531(7594):381–385.

59. Sheahan TP, Sims AC, Leist SR, Schäfer A, Won J, Brown AJ, et al. Comparative therapeutic efficacy of remdesivir and combination lopinavir, ritonavir, and interferon beta against MERS-CoV. *Nat Commun* 2020;11(1):222.

60. Holshue ML, DeBolt C, Lindquist S, Lofy KH, Wiesman J, Bruce H, et al. First case of 2019 novel coronavirus in the United States. *N Engl J Med* 2020;382(10):929–936.

61. Grein J, Ohmagari N, Shin D, Diaz G, Asperges E, Castagna A, et al. Compassionate use of remdesivir for patients with severe Covid-19. *N Engl J Med* 2020;382(24):2327–2336.

62. Gilead Sciences. Study to Evaluate the Safety and Antiviral Activity of Remdesivir (GS-5734™) in Participants With Severe Coronavirus Disease (COVID-19): ClinicalTrials.gov Identifier: NCT04292899; Mar–Dec 2020. Available from: https://clinicaltrials.gov/ct2/show/NCT04292899.

63. Gilead Sciences. Expanded Access Treatment Protocol: Remdesivir (RDV; GS-5734) for the Treatment of SARS-CoV2 (CoV) Infection (COVID-19): Clinicaltrials.gov Identifier NCT04323761; March 2020. Available from: https://clinicaltrials.gov/ct2/show/NCT04323761.

7

The Impact of COVID-19 Pandemic on Patients with Brain Tumours

Ehab Harahsheh, Aimen Vanood, Daniel Gomez Ramos, Marie Grill, and Maciej M Mrugala

Introduction

Central nervous system (CNS) tumours encompass histologically diverse entities with varying prognostic and therapeutic implications. The prevalence of brain tumours has been on the rise in recent decades, resulting in significant morbidity and mortality across all ages [1]. Brain tumours are generally divided into two main categories: primary tumours arising from brain parenchyma or meninges, and secondary tumours related to metastases from systemic malignancies. While metastatic brain tumours are far more common than primary brain tumours, glioma accounts for a good proportion of diagnoses in neuro-oncology practice for the latter group [2]. Treatment of both primary and secondary brain tumours usually requires a multimodal and multidisciplinary approach delivered in a timely fashion to ensure the best possible outcomes in this patient population.

The outbreak of coronavirus disease-19 (COVID-19) and its declaration as a pandemic by the World Health Organization (WHO) in March 2020 had a disruptive and devastating impact on countries, regions, and people's lives worldwide [3]. The pandemic impacted patients' care across all levels and forced health-care systems to quickly adapt, and neuro-oncological practice was no exception. The COVID-19 pandemic imposed significant changes on the care of patients with brain tumours and raised many challenges in maintaining high-quality patient care, ensuring patients, clinical practitioners, and researchers' safety and well-being, and continuing clinical trials and laboratory research projects. Patients with brain tumours usually require frequent visits with their providers and often their neurosurgical oncological procedures, chemotherapy, and radiation therapy sessions are time sensitive. However, in the early months of the pandemic many of these visits and procedures had to be canceled or rescheduled, which created stressful situations for both the patients and their providers [4, 5]. In addition, the COVID-19 outbreak strained health-care systems around the world and created an additional layer of stress and burnout for health-care workers. Clinical trials and basic laboratory research are important aspects for treating patients with brain tumours as they offer possible new therapeutic options in the future for this patient population, but many of these clinical trials and research projects had to be suspended or canceled given the pandemic and financial concerns [6]. In this chapter, we

DOI: 10.1201/9781003362562-8

will attempt to summarise the impact of the COVID-19 outbreak on neuro-oncology practice and describe: (1) the emergence of telemedicine as a potential alternative to in-person visits for managing this patient population, (2) the association between COVID-19 infection and incidence and outcomes of brain tumours, and (3) vaccination rates, safety, and efficacy in brain cancer patients, in addition to suggesting future directions to optimise the care of this patient population beyond the pandemic.

Neuro-Oncology Practice during COVID-19 Pandemic

Tele-Neuro-Oncology

The traditional practice of medicine in general, including neuro-oncology, was significantly affected in the early days of the pandemic. In-person office-based or hospital-based evaluation have been the dominant theme for most patient encounters for many decades, and while telemedicine existed, it failed to gain widespread acceptance among both patients and health-care professionals [7]. Telemedicine, the use of real-time audio or audiovisual technology to deliver healthcare services, is a convenient telecommunication tool that connects a patient to a healthcare provider without the need to be in the same room. The pandemic helped accelerate the widespread use of telemedicine in the neuro-oncology world, and many encounters for patients with brain tumours became virtual and remote with almost universal transition to telemedicine worldwide during the early days of the pandemic. This was further facilitated by loosening the legislative, bureaucratic, and regulatory barriers for reimbursement for telemedicine visits [4, 8]. According to one study, 95% of healthcare professionals in neuro-oncology practice reported that they transitioned to video or telephone visits for some aspects of patient care early during the COVID-19 outbreak [4]. Despite this quick and rapid transition to virtual encounters, the majority of patients with brain tumours and their families were satisfied with telemedicine visits both for medical neuro-oncological encounters, as patients with brain tumours often face logistical challenges surrounding transportation to health-care facilities for follow-up care. It is not uncommon for brain tumour patients to have limited mobility, cognitive dysfunction, and/or vision impairment, and thus transportation can be cost-prohibitive as well as time consuming [9]. Moreover, health-care professionals reported that virtual meetings and video conferences had a positive aspect on their patient care [4, 10]. For example, virtual tumour boards offered new avenues and added another opportunity to help provide multidisciplinary care, discuss challenging cases, and share expertise among providers [10].

Treatment Paradigms for Patients with Brain Tumours during COVID-19 Pandemic

Despite the widespread acceptance of telehealth visits by both health-care professionals and patients with neuro-oncological disorders, neuroimaging, chemotherapy, and radiation therapy sessions still necessitated in-person visits. However, early in the pandemic delays in scheduling, or shortening of these sessions, which occasionally can be time sensitive, were reported [11]. For example, clinical evaluations of patients with asymptomatic or clinically stable meningioma or low-grade meningioma were deferred or delayed at the peak of the pandemic at some centers to minimise the contagion of the virus and prioritise treatment for patients with higher-risk tumours, such as high-grade glioma [11]. Moreover, chemotherapy and myelotoxic medications were avoided whenever possible in frail, elderly patients, especially those with IDH-wild-type unmethylated O6-methylguanine-DNA methyltransferase (MGMT) glioblastoma multiforme (GBM), given the perceived increased risks of immunosuppression and the need for more frequent visits for blood tests and monitoring, therein taking into account the increased risks of acquiring severe acute respiratory syndrome coronavirus 2 (SARS-COV-2) and the limited survival benefits in this patient population [11, 12]. Additionally, consensus recommendations from experts in the neuro-oncology field were made during the pandemic to minimise the generous prescription of corticosteroids to patients with brain tumours as much as possible by using the lowest dose for the shortest period of time to help avoid unnecessary immunosuppression [6]. Institutions and guidelines encouraged the selective use and implementation of hypofractionated radiotherapy for patients with newly diagnosed GBM brain tumour, particularly for the elderly with poor functional status, in order to minimise the risk of exposure for both patients and health-care professionals while not sacrificing clinical outcomes [13].

Surgical practice for these patients was also affected, as many elective surgical procedures were rescheduled, canceled, or modified. One study from multiple neurosurgical units in the UK early in the pandemic reported that at least 10.0% of patients with malignant brain tumours had their surgical plan changed, with a significant proportion having their surgery canceled due to the SARS-CoV-2 outbreak [14]. Institutions and hospitals started triaging their patients for surgical intervention, with a higher priority given to patients with malignant brain tumours or benign brain tumours with severe symptoms while asymptomatic or mildly symptomatic patients with benign tumours, or those whom the expected survival benefit was likely to be marginal, had their surgeries canceled or rescheduled [14–16]. Some surgical interventions for patients with brain tumours often require postprocedural intensive care unit (ICU) monitoring. However, there was a shortage of ICU beds at the peak of the pandemic, limiting their availability for patients with neuro-oncological disorders, which again in turn necessitated cancellation of non-urgent and elective procedures. On the other hand, some close regional centers were able to continue to manage patients with brain tumours at good capacity by implementing a hub-and-spoke system for neuro-oncology where one main hospital was devoted to surgical neuro-oncological cases, chemotherapy, and outpatient visits, while other hospitals were only accepting COVID-19 cases [17]. Additionally, there was an initial avoidance of endonasal approach for brain tumours, given the concern for aerosolisation and potential spread of COVID-19 infection, and some of these procedures were converted to craniotomy [4]. To minimise the potential spread of COVID-19 cases, some institutions applied rigorous protocols to decrease the risk of exposure to the surgical team while others converted to craniotomies over endonasal approach [4, 18].

Research and Clinical Trials during COVID-19 Pandemic

Clinical trials and laboratory-based research are of paramount importance in the care of patients with brain tumours, given the pressing need for new therapeutic options or experimental therapies as progression of brain tumours, especially high-grade tumours, despite standard treatment is not uncommon. Unfortunately, early in the outbreak many ongoing clinical trials for patients with neuro-oncological disorders were held and stopped enrolling patients, new clinical trials were postponed, and laboratory-based research became difficult to conduct [4]. This was in part due to financial and safety concerns, as clinical trials evaluating novel treatments associated with immunosuppression raised ethical concerns regarding whether the potential benefits associated with experimental therapies outweighed the risks of possible immunosuppression during the pandemic [6]. Also, there were concerns that participation in traditionally designed clinical trials could increase the risk of SARS-CoV-2 infection for both participants and research staff. In addition, many institutions shifted resources to manage patients with COVID-19; thus, limiting staff, financial coverage, and resources available to conduct research, and further disrupting the traditional infrastructure of clinical trials [19]. However, workshops and guidelines proposed novel and streamlined means with which to adapt the current methodology of clinical trials to help overcome some of the obstacles and limitations imposed by the SARS-CoV-2 pandemic [20]. Decentralisation of clinical trials, utilisation of teleconferences for trial coordination and data collection, delivery and shipping of investigational products to participants, and increased usage of local centers for imaging and laboratory studies were a few of the suggested examples to mitigate some of the challenges encountered [20, 21].

Psychosocial Impact of the Pandemic on Healthcare Professionals and Researchers

The impact of the pandemic on neuro-oncological practice extended also to the safety and mental wellness of healthcare professionals and researchers caring for this group of patients. Many providers reported an increase in work hours, salary reduction, concerns about job security, and increased fear about their own well-being as well as their families' [4]. Despite the rising trend of mental stress and anxiety among healthcare providers and researchers in this field, institutional psychosocial support availability was limited to some extent. This further exacerbating the psychosocial stress on both healthcare professionals and researchers taking care of this patient population.

COVID-19 Outbreak and Brain Tumours

Incidence and Outcomes of Brain Tumours during the COVID-19 Pandemic

The COVID-19 pandemic and the imposed changes in neuro-oncological practice impacted the care, and to some extent, the outcomes of patients with brain tumours. SARS-CoV-2 has been shown to enter brain cells through interaction with angiotensin-converting enzyme 2 (ACE2) and neuropilin-1 (NRP-1) receptors expressed on the cell membrane of glial and/or neuronal cells [22–24]. In addition, molecular studies have shown that SARS-CoV-2 surface spike(s) glycoprotein may have a binding affinity toward certain receptor proteins expressed on glial/glioma cells, and this can possibly induce glioma tumourigenesis or progression of primary brain tumours [25].

Reports early in the pandemic described a decrease in the number of inpatient consults for new brain tumour diagnoses compared to the pre-pandemic period, suggesting that SARS-CoV-2 infection may have no impact on the incidence of new cases and/or that patients with brain tumours and mild symptoms may have deferred presentation for medical evaluation due to the fear of exposure to COVID-19 [26]. Nevertheless, there have been rising concerns from both patients and healthcare professionals that the changes in neuro-oncological care, especially given more treatment delays, might lead to negative outcomes in this patient population. However, some studies showed no significant difference in mortality rates or tumour control between patients treated before or after the pandemic [26]. For example, one study assessed patients with malignant brain tumours evaluated between 13 March 2020 and 1 May 2020, compared their outcomes to a corresponding control cohort from the same time period in 2019, and reported no significant differences between both groups in terms of mortality or tumour control despite the treatment delays, alterations, and/or cessation and suggested that selective, physician-led delays and adaptations in care may not lead to adverse outcomes [26].

Medical and Psychiatric Complications in Patients with Brain Tumours

Multiple reports showed that patients with cancer, including brain tumours, are at increased risk of developing complications from COVID-19 infection [27–30]. A Dutch report of 30 patients with primary brain tumours who contracted COVID-19 infection reported that 63% of patients had a severe course of COVID-19 infection requiring either hospital admission or leading to fatal outcomes, which is higher when compared to the general population [27]. Another study from Iran demonstrated an increased risk of death from COVID-19 infection in patients with brain tumours compared to other malignancies [28]. Though many factors, such as age and comorbid cardiovascular and pulmonary diseases, may contribute to the increased susceptibility of patients with brain tumours to more deleterious outcomes from COVID-19 infection as seen in the general population, exposure to antineoplastic myelotoxic therapies and cancer-associated immunocompromise have been perceived as more specific potential risk factors in patients with brain tumours [31].

In addition to the medical complications related to COVID-19 infection, patients with brain tumours and their caregivers have experienced significant stress and anxiety during the pandemic. This additional psychosocial stress has been mainly related to the public and private social restrictions experienced by patients and their caregivers during the pandemic and fear of contracting COVID-19 infection, as well as the uncertainty and the concerns for delay in their brain tumour-related appointments or treatment [5, 32]. An increase in anxiety and depression in patients with brain tumours was observed by healthcare professionals, and according to one study approximately 20%–35% of healthcare professionals reported an increase in the frequency of palliative care consults and end-of-life discussions since the beginning of the pandemic [4]. The increase in the frequency of advanced directives and goals of care discussions could be attributed to the emerging focus both of patients with brain tumours as well as their healthcare providers on the importance of quality of life during the pandemic.

COVID-19 Vaccination: Rates, Safety and Efficacy in Patients with Brain Tumours

The advent of multiple approved COVID-19 vaccines and worldwide campaigns for vaccination have contributed to minimising the impact of the pandemic on people, healthcare systems, and countries [33]. Though concerns were raised about the safety and efficacy of vaccines in patients with cancer, given their under-representation in the original trials that led to approval of COVID-19 vaccines and frequent immunosuppression from their treatment regimens, the vast majority of patients with brain tumours and their caregivers received COVID-19 vaccine (85%) according to an international survey of this patient population, with no major side effects reported [34–36]. Another study from Italy of approximately 100 patients with primary brain tumours reported a low rate of adverse events and did not show increased risk for vaccine-induced serious adverse events [35]. Moreover, a study of 17 patients with primary brain tumours who received two doses of BNT162b2 mRNA COVID-19 vaccine had no adverse events [37]. However, this study showed that only 80% of patients with primary brain tumours achieved successful seroconversion following two doses of vaccination, and they had lower IgG antibody titers compared to a healthy control group. Additionally, it reported that corticosteroid treatment can contribute to impaired immunogenicity to COVID-19 vaccines in this patient group [37]. These studies suggest that COVID-19 vaccines are potentially safe without serious adverse reactions in patients with brain tumours, but active immunosuppressive treatment, especially with chronic high-dose corticosteroids, may impair the immunogenicity and lead to suboptimal response to COVID-19 vaccination, similar to other patient populations [38, 39].

Interestingly, a few reports suggested that COVID-19 vaccines may help uncover undiagnosed brain tumours and increase the risk of breakthrough seizures in patients with glioma via induction of inflammatory cascade, as reported patients developed breakthrough seizures or new neurological symptoms shortly after being vaccinated and were found to have neoplastic lesions in the brain parenchyma with surrounding peritumoural edema, which could have been potentiated by the inflammatory response induced by COVID-19 vaccines [40, 41].

Future Directions

Though the COVID-19 pandemic led to unprecedented changes in our medical practice and strained healthcare systems worldwide, it created novel and unique opportunities to adapt and thoughtfully reconsider our current practice and guidelines. The implementation of telemedicine for managing patients with brain tumours helped overcome the limitations of social distancing and shortage of personal protective equipment. It also created new avenues for healthcare delivery for this patient population without necessarily compromising their outcomes, especially given the frequent logistic challenges with transportation for in-person visits. Furthermore, virtual tumour boards offered several advantages during the pandemic, and increased utilisation across and within institutions shall enhance and expand multidisciplinary care, especially for challenging cases. However, this widespread use and implementation of telemedicine was facilitated by loosening legislative, bureaucratic, and reimbursement barriers. To ensure continuous selective utilisation of telemedicine visits for this patient population, governments and institutions need to improve infrastructure and internet connections, especially in rural areas, and continue to improve reimbursement for virtual encounters.

This pandemic emphasised the importance of having early discussions regarding goals of care and advanced directives with patients with brain tumours, especially those with high-grade glioma, considering the limited survival benefits of some of the available treatment options. Therefore, neuro-oncologists should consider alternative options. Offering treatment with limited evidence of efficacy like temozolomide for patients with IDH-wild-type MGMT unmethylated GBM may not always be the best choice, and early palliative care consultation with exploration of other treatment modalities and early clinical trial involvement for interested patients should be strongly considered. In addition, neuro-oncologists should remain mindful of limiting corticosteroid use for patients with brain tumours, in order to minimise the risk of unnecessary immunosuppression in this vulnerable patient population. Documentation of the goals of care discussion and the prognosis for these patients is of paramount importance for our colleagues and societies as it can help with future decision-making processes when calamities occur like the COVID-19 pandemic, during which the shortage of resources raised ethical dilemmas. This pandemic also highlighted the need for healthcare professionals to attend to the psychological well-being of patients with brain tumours and their caregivers, as well as their own.

Finally, current clinical trial design and methodology in the neuro-oncology world need further study and adaptation to ensure continued accrual of patients with brain tumours and minimize the impact of unexpected emergencies akin to the COVID-19 pandemic. Decentralisation of clinical trials and increased usage of virtual visits and local resources for laboratory and imaging studies can help overcome some of these limitations and increase patient recruitment for future trials.

REFERENCES

1. Deorah S, Lynch CF, Sibenaller ZA, Ryken TC. Trends in brain cancer incidence and survival in the United States: Surveillance, epidemiology, and end results program, 1973 to 2001. *Neurosurg Focus* 2006;20(4):E1.
2. Davis ME. Epidemiology and Overview of Gliomas. *Semin Oncol Nurs* 2018;34:420–429. doi: 10.1016/j.soncn.2018.10.001.
3. Haleem A, Javaid M, Vaishya, R. Effects of COVID-19 pandemic in daily life. *Curr Med Res Pract* 2020;10:78–79. doi: 10.1016/j.cmrp.2020.03.011.
4. Mrugala MM, Ostrom QT, Pressley SM, et al. The state of neuro-oncology during the COVID-19 pandemic: A worldwide assessment. *Neurooncol Adv* 2021;3(1):vdab035. doi: 10.1093/noajnl/vdab035.
5. Voisin MR, Oliver K, Farrimond S, et al. Brain tumors and COVID-19: The patient and caregiver experience. *Neurooncol Adv Neurooncol Adv.* 2020;2(1):vdaa104. doi: 10.1093/noajnl/vdaa104.
6. Weller M, Preusser, M. How we treat patients with brain tumour during the COVID-19 pandemic. *ESMO Open* 2020;4(Suppl 2):e000789. doi: 10.1136/esmoopen-2020-000789.
7. Institute of Medicine & Board on Health Care Services. The role of telehealth in an evolving health care environment: Workshop summary. National Academies Press, 2012.

8. Kircher SM, Mulcahy M, Kalyan A, et al. Telemedicine in oncology and reimbursement policy during COVID-19 and beyond. *J Natl Compr Canc Netw* 2020;30:1–7. doi: 10.6004/jnccn.2020.7639.

9. Liu JKC, Kang R, Bilenkin A, et al. Patient satisfaction and cost savings analysis of the telemedicine program within a neuro-oncology department. *J Neurooncol* 2022;160(2):517–525. doi: 10.1007/s11060-022-04173-7.

10. Schäfer N, Bumes E, Eberle F, et al. Implementation, relevance, and virtual adaptation of neuro-oncological tumor boards during the COVID-19 pandemic: A nationwide provider survey. *J Neurooncol* 2021;153:479–485. doi: 10.1007/s11060-021-03784-w.

11. Simonelli M, Franceschi E, Lombardi G. Neuro-oncology during the COVID-19 outbreak: A hopeful perspective at the end of the Italian crisis. *Front Med* 2010;7:594610. doi: 10.3389/fmed.2020.594610.

12. Kamson DO, Grossman SA. The role of temozolomide in patients with newly diagnosed wild-type IDH, unmethylated MGMTp glioblastoma during the COVID-19 pandemic. *JAMA Oncol* 2021;7:675–676. doi: 10.1001/jamaoncol.2020.6732.

13. Noticewala SS, Ludmir EB, Bishop AJ, et al. Radiation for glioblastoma in the era of coronavirus disease 2019 (COVID-19): Patient selection and hypofractionation to maximize benefit and minimize risk. *Adv Radiat Oncol* 2020;5:743–745.

14. Price SJ, Joannides A, Plaha P, et al. Impact of COVID-19 pandemic on surgical neuro-oncology multi-disciplinary team decision making: A national survey (COVID-CNSMDT Study). *BMJ Open* 2020;10:e040898. doi: 10.1016/j.adro.2020.04.040.

15. Hu YJ, Zhang JM, Chen Z. Experiences of practicing surgical neuro-oncology during the COVID-19 pandemic. *J Neurooncol* 2020;148:199–200. doi: 10.1007/s11060-020-03489-6.

16. Hameed NUF, Ma Y, Zhen Z, et al. Impact of a pandemic on surgical neuro-oncology–maintaining functionality in the early phase of crisis. *BMC Surgery* 2021;21(1):40. doi: 10.1186/s12893-021-01055-z.

17. Perin A, Servadei F, DiMeco F; 'Hub and spoke' Lombardy neurosurgery group. May we deliver neuro-oncology in difficult times (e.g. COVID-19)? *J Neurooncol* 2020;148(1):203–205. doi: 10.1007/s11060-020-03496-7.

18. Quillin JW, Oyesiku NM. Status of pituitary surgery during the COVID-19 pandemic. *Neurol India* 2020;68(Supplement):S134–S136. doi: 10.4103/0028-3886.287685.

19. Tan AC, Ashley DM, Khasraw M. Adapting to a pandemic – conducting oncology trials during the SARS-CoV-2 Pandemic. *Clin Cancer Res* 2020;26(13):3100–3103. doi: 10.1158/1078-0432.CCR-20-1364.

20. Lee EQ, Selig W, Meehan C, et al. Report of National Brain Tumor Society roundtable workshop on innovating brain tumor clinical trials: Building on lessons learned from COVID-19 experience. *Neuro Oncol* 2021;23:1252–1260. doi: 10.1093/neuonc/noab082.

21. Yeboa DN, Akinfenwa CA, Nguyen J, et al. Effectively conducting oncology clinical trials during the COVID-19 pandemic. *Adv Radiat Oncol* 2021;6(3):100676. doi: 10.1016/j.adro.2021.100676.

22. Baig AM, Khaleeq A, Ali U, Syeda H. Evidence of the COVID-19 virus targeting the CNS: Tissue distribution, host-virus interaction, and proposed neurotropic mechanisms. *ACS Chem Neurosci* 2020;11(7):995–998. doi: 10.1021/acschemneuro.0c00122.

23. Chekol Abebe E, Mengie Ayele T, Tilahun Muche Z, Asmamaw Dejenie T. Neuropilin 1. A novel entry factor for SARS-CoV-2 infection and a potential therapeutic target. *Biologics* 2021;15:143–152. doi: 10.2147/BTT.S307352.

24. Lei J, Liu Y, Xie T, Yao G, Wang G, Diao B, Song J. Evidence for residual SARS-CoV-2 in glioblastoma tissue of a convalescent patient. *Neuroreport* 2021;32(9):771–775. doi: 10.1097/WNR.0000000000001654.
25. Khan I, Hatiboglu MA. Can COVID-19 induce glioma tumorogenesis through binding cell receptors? *Med Hypotheses* 2020;144:110009. doi: 10.1016/j.mehy.2020.110009.
26. Norman S, Ramos A, Giantini Larsen A et al. Impact of the COVID-19 pandemic on neuro-oncology outcomes. *J Neurooncol* 2021;154(3):375–381. doi: 10.1007/s11060-021-03838-z.
27. de Joode K, Taal W, Snijders TJ et al. Patients with primary brain tumors and COVID-19: A report from the Dutch oncology COVID-19 consortium. *Neuro Oncol* 2022;24:326–328. doi: 10.1093/neuonc/noab258.
28. Fazilat-Panah D, Fallah Tafti H, Rajabzadeh Y, et al. Clinical characteristics and outcomes of COVID-19 in 1294 new cancer patients: Single-center, prospective cohort study from Iran. *Cancer Invest* 2022;40(6):505–515. doi: 10.1080/07357907.2022.2075376.
29. Williams M, Mi E, Le Calvez K, et al. Estimating the risk of death from COVID-19 in adult cancer patients. *Clin Oncol* 2021;2021(33):e172–e179. doi: 10.1016/j.clon.2020.10.021.
30. Kuderer NM, Choueiri TK, Shah DP, et al. Clinical impact of COVID-19 on patients with cancer (CCC19): A cohort study. *Lancet* 2020;395:1907–1918. doi: 10.1016/S0140-6736(20)31187-9.
31. Bernhardt D, Wick W, Weiss SE, et al. Neuro-oncology management during the COVID-19 pandemic with a focus on WHO grades III and IV gliomas. *Neuro Oncol* 2020;22:928–935. doi: 10.1093/neuonc/noaa113.
32. Binswanger J, Kohl C, Behling F, et al. Neuro-oncological patients' and caregivers' psychosocial burden during the COVID-19 pandemic – a prospective study with qualitative content analysis. *Psychooncology* 2021;30:1502–1513. doi: 10.1002/pon.5713.
33. Watson OJ, Barnsley G, Toor J, Hogan AB, Winskill P, Ghani AC. Global impact of the first year of COVID-19 vaccination: A mathematical modelling study. *Lancet Infect Dis* 2022;22:1293–1302. doi: 10.1016/S1473-3099(22)00320-6.
34. Voisin MR, Oliver K, Farrimond S, et al. Brain tumor patients and COVID-19 vaccines: Results of an international survey. *Neurooncol Adv* 2022;4(1):vdac063. doi: 10.1093/noajnl/vdac063.
35. Tanzilli A, Pace A, Ciliberto G, et al. COV-BT Ire study: Safety and efficacy of the BNT162b2 mRNA COVID-19 vaccine in patients with brain tumors. *Neurol Sci* 2022; 43, 3519–3522. doi: 10.1007/s10072-022-06054-3.
36. Baden LR, El Sahly HM, Essink B, et al. Efficacy and safety of the mRNA-1273 SARS-CoV-2 vaccine. *N Engl J Med* 2021;384:403–416. doi: 10.1056/NEJMoa2035389.
37. Massarweh A, Tschernichovsky R, Stemmer A, et al. Immunogenicity of the BNT162b2 mRNA COVID-19 vaccine in patients with primary brain tumors: A prospective cohort study. *J Neurooncol* 2022;156(3):483–489. doi: 10.1007/s11060-021-03911-7.
38. Rabinowich L, Grupper A, Baruch R, et al. Low immunogenicity to SARS-CoV-2 vaccination among liver transplant recipients. *J Hepatol* 2021;75:435–438. doi: 10.1016/j.jhep.2021.04.020.
39. Ferri C, Ursini F, Gragnani L, et al. Impaired immunogenicity to COVID-19 vaccines in autoimmune systemic diseases. High prevalence of non-response in different patients' subgroups. *J Autoimmun* 2021;125:102744. doi: 10.1016/j.jaut.2021.102744.

40. Einstein EH, Shahzadi A, Desir L, et al. New-onset neurologic symptoms and related neuro-oncologic lesions discovered after COVID-19 vaccination: Two neurosurgical cases and review of post-vaccine inflammatory responses. *Cureus* 2021;13(6):e15664. doi: 10.7759/cureus.15664.
41. Shah T, Figuracion KC, Schteiden B, Graber, J. Breakthrough seizures after COVID-19 vaccines in patients with glioma (P4-9.005). *Neurology* 2022;98(18 Suppl).

8

SARS-CoV-2 Infection and Colorectal Cancer: Potential Implication

Gabriella Marfe, Stefania Perna, and Giovanna Mirone

Introduction

After the first report of severe acute respiratory syndrome coronavirus 2 (SARS-CoV-2) at the end December 2019, this virus had infected about 560 million individuals around the world by the middle of February 2021 [1, 2]. On January 4, 2023, data revealed that since the start of the outbreak, 655,689,115 individuals have been diagnosed with severe acute respiratory syndrome coronavirus 2 (SARS-CoV-2) infection globally, and 6,671,624 deaths have been reported by the WHO (https://covid19.who.int/). Based on the scientific literature, SARS-CoV-2 is a positive-sense single-stranded RNA virus that can infect humans and spread easily through binding between spike protein and the human angiotensin-converting enzyme (ACE2) receptor with proteolytic cleavage of ACE2 by transmembrane serine protease [3]. After binding, the enzyme transforms angiotensin I into angiotensin 1–9, which in turn, generates angiotensin 1–7 that reacts with the MAS receptor (a G protein-coupled receptor). Previous studies have suggested that the binding of the SARS-CoV-2 spike protein to ACE2 allows both the viral entry and suppression of ACE2 expression. In this way it would be possible the internalisation and shedding of ACE2 from the cell surface, which in turn could lead to increased levels of angiotensin II. After this process, this molecule binds to its receptor AT1 (angiotensin II receptor type 1) and causes an strong inflammatory response in the lungs, inducing direct parenchymal injury. Other studies identified that the ACE2 receptor and transmembrane protease serine 2 (TMPRSS2) were involved in viral binding to the cell and subsequent entry. Moreover, the spike protein can interact with different receptors and proteases in other tissues [4, 5]. However, the receptor of SARS-CoV-2 also is widely distributed in other parts of the body and for this reason, the virus can harm other body organs. A high prevalence of SARS-CoV-2 infection was observed in cancer patients who can develop severer symptoms, mainly because of their compromised immune systems and the malignancy state [6, 7]. In a study, Wang et al. [8] have observed that the prevalence of infection among cancer patients was 24.7% in lung cancer, 20.5% in colorectal cancer, and 13.0% in breast cancer, suggesting an additional risk to these patients [8]. Furthermore, the pooled data showed that there was an increased risk for COVID-19 infection in CRC patients (95% CI 0.13–0.29, $p \leq 0.001$) [8]. In another analysis, Aznab [9] estimated the prevalence and determinants of symptomatic COVID-19 infection in 279 cancer patients within 90 days in Kermanshah City, Iran. Their data reported the COVID-19 infection in 72 CRC, 11 cases of lung cancer, 5 brain tumours, and 12 ovarian cancers [9]. Another research study found that COVID 19–positive cancer patients had a higher risk of severe/critical disease and mortality than non-cancer patients [10]. The ACE2 receptor plays a critical role in the pathogenesis of COVID-19, and in this regard, the authors in two studies have tried to understand the susceptibility of cancer patients to SARS-CoV-2 infection and disease outcome considering ACE2 expression levels in cancer tissues and related bioinformatic assays [11, 12]. In the first study, Zhang et al. have observed that patients with non-small cell lung cancer were more susceptible to COVID-19 because of upregulated ACE2 expression in tumour tissues [11]. In the second paper, Zhou et al. also have noted that ACE2 expression levels were elevated in uterine corpus endometrial carcinoma and kidney renal papillary cell carcinoma tissues, and such upregulation was positively correlated with survival outcomes. Furthermore, they suggested that SARS-CoV-2 infection can have a strong impact on these patients, thereby worsening their clinical outcomes through immune-related processes [12]. Many clinical case reports showed that some patients infected with SARS-CoV-2 experienced digestive symptoms [13–15], such as abdominal pain, diarrhoea, appetite loss, nausea, vomiting, and blood glucose disorders. At the beginning, patients affected by this disease did not report significant symptoms involving the digestive system and only 2.6% had diarrhoea and 2% had chronic diseases of the liver [16]. During the pandemic, more and more patients suffered digestive system symptoms such as diarrhoea, anorexia, nausea, vomiting, abdominal discomfort, and gastrointestinal bleeding. Several potential pathways seemed involved in the development of gastrointestinal problems. These include virus-induced cytopathic impacts through ACE2, immune-mediated inflammatory cytokine storm, and the function of the gut-lung axis as well as drug-related harm. These pathways can also contribute to sepsis and acute respiratory distress syndrome (ARDS), which are the leading causes of death in COVID-19 patients. Different studies described symptoms such as diarrhoea, reported with a rate ranging from 2.0 to 47.9% in COVID-19 patients [16–21]. Even though the first COVID-19 clinical article reported that only 1 in 38 patients had diarrhoea [16], the frequency of diarrhoea is usually greater in later stages. A cohort study carried out with 73 COVID-19 patients reported that diarrhoea was observed in up to 35.6% of patients [20]. Similarly, the incidence of diarrhoea was up to 47.9% in a cohort of 305 patients reported by Fang et al [18]. Furthermore, Wang et al reported an incidence of up to 39.9% and Fang et al reported 33.1% [18, 19]. According to data, patients with nausea account for 1.0–19.3% [17–21]. Moreover, in their study, Xiao et al [19] did not find substantial mucosal epithelial harm of the oesophagus, stomach, duodenum, and rectum using H&E (hematoxylin and eosin) staining. Occasionally, they observed lymphocyte infiltration in the oesophageal squamous epithelium. Moreover, the virus nucleocapsid protein was found in the gastric, duodenal, and rectal glandular cytoplasm. This means that SARS-CoV-2 could directly target gastrointestinal cells, especially gastric and intestinal epithelial cells, leading to inflammatory reactions. Lin et al. [22] examined 95 COVID-19–contaminated cases and performed endoscopic examinations on the gastrointestinal cases. The authors found the virus in various sections of the gastrointestinal tract. In addition, Xiao et al. [19] detected that about 20% of patients were positive for virus in their stool, even after the respiratory tract was cleared of the virus. These studies demonstrated the presence of SARS-CoV-2 in COVID-19 patients, which means that gastrointestinal symptoms could be correlated with viral infections in patients with COVID-19. In nearly half of the COVID-19 patients with digestive symptoms, viral RNA can be detected in their stool for determining the diagnosis and transmission [23]. In this regard, a research study showed that SARS-CoV-2 was able to enter cells through the ACE2 receiver [24]. Moreover, another study has suggested a possible mechanism for the digestive symptoms in COVID-19 patients. ACE2 expression on the small intestine surface cells can mediate viral invasion and expansion, triggering gastrointestinal inflammation [25]. SARS-CoV-2 invades intestinal cells expressing ACE2, causing malabsorption, intestinal disorders, activation of the enteric nervous system, and, ultimately, diarrhoea. Interestingly, a previous study on other coronaviruses found that human intestinal epithelial cells' high sensitivity to coronavirus increases their replicative capacity [26]. These results suggested that the SARS-CoV-2 virus was transmitted among patients with COVID-19 through the fecal–oral route [13–15, 27]. Therefore, gastrointestinal infection and potential fecal–oral transmission can last even after viral clearance from the respiratory tract [20], which makes gastroenterology clinical management more difficult during cases of SARS-CoV-2 infection [28]. In addition, recent studies have reported that COVID-19 patients lose commensal taxa of the gut microbiome during hospitalisation [29–31]. Differences in gut bacterial populations relative to healthy controls were observed in all COVID-19 patients, but most strongly in patients who were treated with antibiotics during their hospitalisation. Most recently, COVID-19 patients treated with broad spectrum antibiotics at admission were shown to have increased susceptibility to multi-drug–resistant infections and nearly double the mortality rate from septic shock [32, 33]. Furthermore, although initially estimated to be low (6.5%) [34], more recent studies have detected bacterial secondary infections in as much as 12–14% of COVID-19 patients [35, 36]. However, the causal direction of the relationship between disease symptoms and gut bacterial populations is not yet clear. Moreover, increasing data have reported the correlation of the immune state in colon cancer with the patient's prognosis [37], and for this reason it is possible to suppose colon cancer patients might be very vulnerable to SARS-CoV-2 infection by associating the elevated expression levels of the ACE2 in these patients and its role in SARS-CoV-2 pathogenesis. Although further validation of clinical data is needed, these results can play a crucial role in patients with clinically mild or moderate COVID-19 with a diagnosis of colorectal cancer, and it is necessarily of particular attention because of a possible longer course of disease or a higher risk of severe infection probability.

Search Strategy and Selection Criteria

We considered scientific articles from online sources, journals, and media reports. The literature was collected from March 2020 (at the begining of the first wave of COVID-19 pandemic) until the end of this study (July 2022). We used different databases such as Scopus (scopus.com), Web of Science (webofscience.com), Google scholar, and PubMed Central (PMC). In this process we used different keywords such as "COVID-19" or "SARS-CoV-2" from the end of 2019 until July 2022 to develop the right search criteria. In addition, other search keywords were "colorectal cancer, ACE and TMPRSS2". Then, we chose only articles in English language and analysed them considering the selected keywords. The final reference list was prepared on the basis of relevance to the broad scope of this chapter.

The Impact of SARS-CoV-2 Infection on Gut Microbiome Dysbiosis and Colorectal Cancer

Multiple studies showed that cancer patients had a higher risk of infection and adverse events when compared with patients without cancer and it could be attributed it to systemic immunosuppression in cancer patients [38]. For example, He et al. [39] believed that COVID-19 infection could occur prior to symptom onset in 44% patients. For this reason, during colonoscopy or colorectal cancer surgery, it is necessary to avoid aerosol contamination from the creation of laparoscopic pneumoperitoneum, or intestinal secretions and fecal contamination from the disposal of intestinal tract and tumours, even in asymptomatic patients. Therefore, it is necessary to increase the strict infection control through prevention measures applied during gastrointestinal tumour surgery. A limited case series from China studies showed that some COVID-19 patients had decreased Lactobacillus and Bifidobacterium microbial dysbiosis [40]. Nevertheless, previous research has shown that ACE2 can adjust intestinal microbe homeostasis through amino acids [41], For example, strong microbiota may ferment to generate fatty acids (SCFAs), and most SCFAs are metabolised. Unmetabolised SCFAs promote the development of naive CD4 + T cells to regulate cells in the peripheral circulation and bone marrow. Thus, immune response in the lungs would be impaired if the intestinal microbiota stability is disrupted. Furthermore, cytokines and inflammatory cells increase in COVID-19 patients and were associated with sepsis and ARDS complications [42, 43]. Studies have shown that cytokine storms can be inhibited by butyric acid provided by the intestinal microbiota [44].Therefore, the incidence of sepsis and ARDS may be minimised by the intestinal microbiota, both of which have a high mortality risk in COVID-19. Moreover, some researchers consider the connection between sepsis and intestinal microbiota disorders to be jointly promoted [45]. This indicates that disease of the gastrointestinal microbiota causes the development of sepsis, and in effect, the stable structure of the intestinal microbiota is disrupted, followed by the creation of a destructive cycle. Furthermore, intestinal tissue or tumour specimens should be handled in a safe manner to reduce the risk of transmission caused by intestinal infection and to prevent nosocomial infections. In this regard, Qian et al described a case report of a patient with fever and cough after 3 days postoperatively. This patient tested positive for COVID-19 on day 7, and he was discharged from the hospital after 41 days. The RNA of SARS-CoV-2 was found in the surgically resected rectal specimens but not in samples collected 37 days after discharge. Furthermore, typical coronavirus virions were detected in rectal tissue of surgical specimens (positive to RNA of SARS-CoV-2) under electron microscopy. Moreover, abundant lymphocytes and macrophages (some were SARS-CoV-2 positive) infiltrating the lamina propria were observed with no significant mucosal damage. This study reported the evidence of active SARS-CoV-2 replication in a patient's rectum during the incubation period, which might explain SARS-CoV-2 fecal–oral transmission [46]. Other clinical studies reported that SARS-CoV-2 can enter into the gastrointestinal system through ACE2 where it is highly expressed along with TMPRSS2 [47, 48]. Furthermore, adaptor-associated protein kinase 1 – also known as AP2-associated protein kinase 1 (AAK1) – facilitates the passage of viruses into cells along with TMPRSS2. Many findings showed that ACE-2 expression level was upregulated in a wide variety of adenocarcinomas, including GI tract carcinoma. In a study,

Bernardi et al. found that MasR and ACE-2 expression were both increased in colon adenocarcinoma cells as compared to controls or non-neoplastic colon mucosa resected 5 cm from tumour borders [49]. In accordance with these data, in another study, the authors observed that expression levels for ACE2, TMPRSS2, and AAK1 were positively associated in colon cells using Database of Gene expression profiling interactive analysis. Therefore, they suggested this virus could increase complications in patients with colon cancer [50]. Another interesting study found that ACE2 and TMPRSS2 were highly expressed in colonic tissue in younger patients with greater TMPRSS2 expression in females. Specifically, the authors found that ACE2 and TMPRSS2 expression were more upregulated in human colorectal tumour or normal tissue samples when compared with human tumour or normal tissue samples of lung, esophagus, stomach, and liver through bulk RNA-sequencing profiling. Furthermore, they observed that the ACE2 and TMPRSS2 expression levels in human tumour and normal colorectal tissues were upregulated above all in colorectal epithelial cells through bulk and single-cell RNA-sequencing datasets. In addition, they examined both COVID-19–positive patients with colorectal cancer and COVID-19 positive patients without cancer. In this regard, they found that cancer patients had lymphopenia and higher respiratory rates and hypersensitive C-reactive protein levels when compared with COVID-19–positive patients without cancer. The data indicate that patients with colorectal cancer may be at high risk of SARS-CoV-2 infection and severe disease [51]. In another study, it was observed that the expression levels of ACE2 and TMPRSS2 proteins were higher in colorectal cancer tissues than normal tissues using Gene Expression Profiling Interactive Analysis (GEPIA). In addition, the expression levels of ACE2 and TMPRSS2 expression did not depend on different clinical stages of colorectal cancer [52]. In another paper, the authors evaluated gene expression of ACE2 and TMPRSS2 across 31 types of tumours. Specifically, they observed overexpression of ACE2 and TMPRSS2 in colorectal cancer including colon adenocarcinoma (COAD) and rectum adenocarcinoma (READ). In this regard, they found an association between an upregulated gene expression and decreased DNA methylation levels. The authors suggested that care management of colorectal cancer patients should be improved during the COVID-19 pandemic [53]. According to these data, in another article, the authors found that the methylation status of the ACE2 promoter in colon adenocarcinoma was significantly reduced compared with matched normal tissues. Thus, DNA methylation may be implicated in the molecular mechanism of the ACE2 gene overexpression in tumour tissues and colon cancer's pathogenesis. Furthermore, the authors showed that ACE2 gene expression was associated with the immune cell infiltration levels in patients with colon adenocarcinoma. For this reason, they suggested that these patients are more likely to be infected with SARS-CoV-2 and experience severe injuries [54]. In light of this, it can be important to underline that SARS-CoV-2 infection induces cytokine storm, which in turn causes systemic inflammation, various organ dysfunction, reduced amount of natural killer cells and T cells, and dysregulated activation of neutrophils, monocytes, and macrophages. In particular, these neutrophils produce different substances such as protein and DNA web-like structures, which are also known as neutrophil extracellular traps (NETs). Different studies reported that the strong proinflammatory cytokine release and NET can induce both the dormant cancer cells (DCCs) and metastasis through several processes such as (1) strong proinflammatory cytokines release such as interleukin 6 (IL-6) can active NF-κβ in both immune and non-immune cells which can lead to increased cancer cell proliferation and pro-metastatic microenvironment induction, (2) lipopolysaccharide-induced lung infection can reactivate both epithelial-mesenchymal transition (EMT) and metastasis of breast DCCs, (3) COVID-19 can induce hypoxia and respiratory distress causing DCCs generation, drug resistance, EMT, and stemness, and (4) NET-related proteases can damage laminin and induce integrin pathway in lung-resident DCCs, thereby cause proliferation and lung metastasis [55–58]. Moreover, numerous studies reported that ACE2 can be involved in development of metastasis. In this regard, deregulation ACE may cause metastasis development in breast cancer, or a low expression level of ACE2 as was associated with lymph node metastasis in squamous cell carcinoma of the gallbladder [59–62]. Therefore, the authors suggest that the virus could active metastasis in COAD patients through cytokine storm-related mechanisms and probable downregulation of ACE2 in their tumour tissues [54]. In another paper, Zhong et al. [63] studied surgical samples derived from a patient with colon cancer and COVID-19 and two tissue microarrays comprising 103 colorectal cancer and 108 enterocyte cases pathologically. The data showed that SARS-CoV-2 nucleocapsid antibody was positively expressed in colon cancer tissues, while the ACE2 was highly expressed in both colorectal cancer tissue microarray and tumour tissue of the patient with a positive rate around 93.2%. Finally, this patient presented a very low immune homeostasis, due to the decrease in TIA + and Granzyme B+ (GrB) CD8 + T cell proportion and the increase in PD-1 + CD8 + T cell proportion. In summary, the authors speculate that these three factors may have contributed significantly to infection risk and severity in the patient [63]. Another Italian study [64] described three patients with metastatic colorectal cancer (mCRC) who were infected by SARS-CoV-2. The authors observed a decrease of disease burden during COVID-19 (coronavirus disease 2019 (COVID-19) course. The authors speculated that the virus might infect ACE-2/NRP-1-expressing colon-cancer cells, causing an immune response against these cells. Moreover, SARS-CoV-2 the binding between SARS-CoV-2 and ACE-2/NRP-1 in CRC cells might lead to cytokine release and an increased number of immune cells in the tumour microenvironment (TME). Furthermore, cross-reactivity with viral antigens might play a crucial role in T (via T-cell receptor interactions) or NK (natural killer) lymphocytes [via ADCC (antibody-dependent cellular cytotoxicity)] activation against CRC cells. However, the natural immunity lymphocytes (including NK cells), which are non-major-histocompatibility-complex restricted, are able to quickly target with transformed or antibody-targeted cells (killing via ADCC). Furthermore in the same study, the authors observed another 60 mCRC patients: seven patients, not included in this report, developed COVID-19 and recovered from it in a median time of 34 days. Then, four patients displayed undetectable response (IgG < 0.04 U/ml) and three showed IgG 0.8, 1.1, 3.6 U/ml [64]. However, these patients did not show tumour burden reduction [64]. Based on these data, Ottaiano et al. performed follow-up clinical research about the patients as well as genetic characterisation of their primary tumours through the TruSigt™Oncology 500 Next Generation Sequencing test targeting 523 cancer relevant genes. The authors found that patients 1 and 2 had the greatest anti-SARS-CoV-2 IgG titres, and in addition had a common mutation in BARD1 gene (p.Val507Met) [65]. In this regard, the authors hypothesise potential interactions between genetic background and components of the immune response to SARS-CoV-2 infection that could be responsible of unexpected rare mCRC shrinkage [65]. These findings may contribute to generate hypotheses on the infection mechanism of the SARS-CoV- 2 virus and the multiple aspects of a composite antiviral immune response in cancer [64, 65]. In this context, we should remember that CRC is characterised by many alterations in the bacterial makeup of the GI microbiota and for this reason dysbiosis plays a crucial role in the development of CRC [66, 67]. Although the microbiota's role in the central processing of complex signals of colorectal carcinogenesis is partially understood, the relationship between virus and the microbial dysbiosis of the GI in this kind of cancer is very complicated and it is unclear. Recent studies have reported that microbial dysbiosis in the lung and GI microbiota induced by SARS-CoV-2 might activate its pathogenic process [68] (Table 8.1) GI microbiota dysbiosis has been associated with sporadic CRC as well as respiratory disorders, including chronic obstructive pulmonary disease [68]. At this point we should ask ourselves two questions: (1) can

TABLE 8.1

The SARS-CoV-2 Infection is Correlated with Significant Changes in the Composition and Function of Gut Microbiome with Several Biological Effects

Gut microbes involved in SARS-CoV-2 infection	Biological effects	References
Coprobacillus, C. ramous, C. hathewayi, B. nordii, A viscosus, Erisipelotrichacea bacterium 2_2-44A	The stability of gut immune homestasis and regulation of inflammation are correlated with the reduction of these bacteria. In addition, Coprobacillus is involved in the upregulation of colonic expression of ACE2 in the murine gut.	[29]
Collinsella aerofaciens, C. tanakaei, Streptococcus infantis, Morganella morganii, C hathewayi, E avium	Increase of these opportunistic pathogens activates both gut inflammation and dysbiosis.	[77]
Streptococcus, Costridium, Peptostreptococcus, Fusobacterium, Citrobacter	The increase of these bacteria induces a high concentration of inflammatory cytokines (IL-8) in the intestine and the development of cytokine storm.	[74]
Faecalibacterium prausnitzii, lostridium butyricum, Clostridium leptum, Eubacterium rectale, Lactobacillus, Bifidobacterium	These bacteria produce butyrate, regulate immunity and integrity of epithelial carrier through IL2, and promote immune system tolerance.	[76]
Faecalibacterium prausnitzii, Alistipes onderdonkii, Bacteroides dorei, acteroides taiotaomicron, Bacteroides massiliensis, Bacteroides ovatus	Anti-inflammatory effects, immune regulation. *B. dorei* downregulates the expression of ACE2 in the gut.	[29]
Bacteroides, Roseburia, Faecalibacterium, Coprococcus, Parabacteroides, Bilophila, Citrobacter	The increase of these bacteria induces a high concentration of of inflammatory cytokines (IL-8) in the intestine and the development of cytokine storm.	[74]
Parabacteroides merdae, Bacteroides stercoris, Alistipes onderdonkii, Lachnospiraceae bacterium 1_1_57FAA	This kind of bacteria produce SCFAs to regulate immunity and integrity of epithelial barrier and immune homeostasis. Specifically, *Bacteroides stercoris* downregulates the expression of ACE2 in the gut.	[77]

colorectal cancer patients with dysbiosis of gut microbiota have an increased possibility to be infected by SARS-CoV-2 and (2) might a long-lasting impact of SARS-CoV-2 on gut dysbiosis cause an increase of CRC diagnosis or worsening the health condition in those already suffered. A pan-cancer study showed that ACE2 and TMPRSS2 had a higher expression level than normal tissue and digestive organs (both tumour and normal samples) than in tumour tissues [69]. In particular, one study demonstrated that colon epithelial cells had high expression levels of ACE2 that strengthened viral replication of SARS-CoV-2, leading to a gut barrier dysfunction [70]. Furthermore, the host proteases to process both spike and S2 domain exposure are present, including TMPRSS2 and TMPRSS4 [71]. For this reason, the local inflammation in the gut epithelia in association with the systemic inflammation derived from the respiratory infection from SARS-CoV-2 can lead to a significant impact on resident gut microbiota leading to dysbiosis. In this regard, this dysbiosis can influence carcinogenesis and the progression of colorectal cancer [29, 72], since this kind of gut microbiota is not able to signal in a correct manner to the presence of bacterial metabolic products in distal tissues. In addition, viral infections in association with systemic inflammation lead to an increased dysbiosis in the symbiotic microbiome within the host [73]. Different studies have demonstrated that COVID-19 induced a dysbiotic microbiota of the gut in patients [74–76]. Furthermore, COVID-19 patients had persistent alterations in the fecal microbiome association with the increase of opportunistic pathogens and depletion of beneficial commensals during hospitalisation. Decreased symbionts and gut dysbiosis could persist after clearance of SARS-CoV-2 and resolution of respiratory symptoms. In addition, one study [77] indicated that dysbiosis occurred in COVID-19 patients, and changes in the gut microbial community were associated with disease severity and hematological parameters. Another study highlighted that some patients had an active viral infection up to 6 days after clearance of SARS-CoV-2 from respiratory samples [78]. In these patients, the authors found a high presence of SARS-CoV-2 in fecal samples in association with abundances of bacterial species such as *Collinsella aerofaciens*, *Collinsella tanakaei*, *Streptococcus infantis*, and *Morganella morganii* [78]. All these studies showed that COVID-19 patients had both a reduction of bacterial diversity in the gut and acute and long-term metabolic effects [77, 78]. Furthermore, in these patients, the presence of butyrate-producing bacteria, such as *Faecalibacterium prausnitzii*, *Clostridium butyricum*, *Clostridium leptum*, and *Eubacterium rectale* may help discriminate critically ill patients from patients that have a more moderate disease state [79]. Moreover, a low-to-no SARS-CoV-2 infectivity was associated with high abundances of SCFA (short-chain fatty acids)-producing bacteria (*Parabacteroides merdae*, *Bacteroides stercoris*, *Alistipes onderdonkii*, and *Lachnospiraceae bacterium* 1_1_57FAA) in fecal samples [78]. Importantly, butyrate-producing bacteria play a critical role in maintaining gut barrier integrality [80]. In addition, SCFAs are involved in the signaling pathway for IL-22, which, in turn, are able to preserve gut and lung epithelial barrier integrity [80]. Moreover, butyrate and SCFAs are regulators of the inflammation produced by macrophages in the intestine and can induce the Warburg effect, which causes an altered metabolism in the neoplastic cells [81]. Furthermore, another bacterium known as *Fusobacterium nucleatum* was found in severe COVID-19 cases; it was able to colonise colon mucus causing a mucosal inflammation, causing immunosuppression [82]. This bacterium recruits tumour-infiltrating immune cells, thus producing a pro-inflammatory microenvironment, which promotes colorectal neoplasia progression.

In addition, it was able to potentiate CRC development through different receptors such as toll-like receptor 2 (TLR2)/toll-like receptor 4 (TLR4) signaling and microRNA (miRNA)-21 expression [82]. Interestingly, one study reported that COVID-19–positive patients had important changes in their fecal fungal microbiomes (mycobiome) (including *Candida albicans, Candida auris*, and *Aspergillus flavus*). In addition, the authors found two respiratory-associated fungal pathogens, *A. flavus* and *Aspergillus niger* in fecal samples from a subset of patients with COVID-19, even after clearance of SARS-CoV-2 from nasopharyngeal samples and resolution of respiratory symptoms [79]. Many papers described prolonged effects after infection, characterised by immune dysregulation and gastrointestinal symptoms, thus impacting the status of the patient's microbiome [83–85]. The possible relationship between SARS-CoV-2 infection and intestinal flora dysbiosis should be validated in a larger cohort considering subgroups at different stages of the disease. Moreover, a study based on the GMrepo database analysed the gut microbiota of both 1,374 patients with colorectal neoplasms and 27,329 healthy people. Additionally, the authors examined feces samples from 12 patients with colorectal cancer and 8 healthy people in Xiangya hospital for metabolomic analysis. They detected an increased presence of Blautia and Ruminococcus in colorectal patients who might be more susceptible to the severity of COVID-19 than healthy people [86]. In this regard, the author concluded that a gut microbiota imbalance is a risk factor of COVID-19 mortality and gut microbiota may provide a new therapeutic avenue for colorectal cancer patients [86].

Conclusion and Future Directions

Today, it is necessary to elucidate the long-term effect of COVID-19 already on mortality and morbidity of the respective patients. The global COVID-19 pandemic caused by SARS-CoV-2 significantly affected patients with different types of cancer worldwide. As discussed previously, patients with CR cancers can be more susceptible to SARS-CoV-2 infection when compared to the general population due to higher expression of ACE-2 and TMPRSS2, which can serve as an entry route for SARS-CoV-2 into target cells. Many papers described prolonged effects after infection, characterised by immune dysregulation and gastrointestinal symptoms, thus impacting the status of the patient's microbiome. In contrast to the dysbiosis leading to colorectal cancer, some studies reported that this cancer in some patients could regress in response to viral infection, known as oncolytic therapy. The gut microbiota plays a crucial role both SARS-CoV-2 infection and CRC development because of an increased expression of genes involved in the inflammatory response with gut barrier dysfunction. Furthermore, changes induced by SARS-CoV-2 infection may further aggravate CRC progression through increased expression of cancer markers, tumour immunosuppression, and the induction of inflammation, leading to gut barrier disruption and worsening CRC progression. However, more knowledge is necessary to understand how SARS-CoV-2 can impact colon progression. Today, there are not enough studies on the association between SARS-CoV-2 and the host microbiome, or virus and niche environments, such as the gut microbiota and its relation to colorectal cancer. More research is necessary to understand in which way SARS-CoV-2 infection influences the gut microbiota and colorectal progression.

CREDIT AUTHORSHIP CONTRIBUTION STATEMENT

Gabriella Marfe: Conceptualisation, formal analysis, methodology, visualisation, software, writing – original draft, – review, and editing. **Stefania Perna**: Writing – original draft, – review, and editing. **Giovanna Mirone**: Writing – review and editing.

DECLARATION OF COMPETING INTEREST

The authors declare that they have no known competing financial interests or personal relationships that could have appeared to influence the work reported in this chapter.

ACKNOWLEDGMENT

This chapter was not supported by a grant.

REFERENCES

1. Zhou P, Yang X, Wang X, Hu B, Zhang L, Zhang W, Si HR, Zhu Y, Li B, Huang CL, Chen HD, Chen J, Luo Y, Guo H, Jiang RD, Liu MQ, Chen Y, Shen XR, Wang X, Zheng XS, Zhao K, Chen QJ, Deng F, Liu LL, Yan B, Zhan FX, Wang YY, Xiao GF, Shi ZL. A pneumonia outbreak associated with a new coronavirus of probable bat origin. *Nature* 2020;579:270–273. doi: 10.1038/s41586-020-2951-z.
2. World Health Organization: WHO coronavirus (COVID-19) dashboard. (2022). Accessed: May 13, 2022 from https://covid19.who.int.
3. Kuba K, Imai Y, Penninger JM. Multiple functions of angiotensin-converting enzyme 2 and its relevance in cardiovascular diseases. *Circ J* 2013;77:301–308. doi: 10.1253/circj.cj-12-1544.
4. Glowacka I, Bertram S, Müller MA, Allen P, Soilleux E, Pfefferle S, Steffen I, Tsegaye TS, He Y, Gnirss K, Niemeyer D, Schneider H, Drosten C, Pöhlmann S. Evidence that TMPRSS2 activates the severe acute respiratory syndrome coronavirus spike protein for membrane fusion and reduces viral control by the humoral immune response. *J Virol* 2011;85(9):4122–4134. doi: 10.1128/JVI.02232-10.
5. Matsuyama S, Nagata N, Shirato K, Kawase M, Takeda M, Taguchi F. Efficient activation of the severe acute respiratory syndrome coronavirus spike protein by the transmembrane protease TMPRSS2. *J Virol* 2010;84(24):12658–12664. doi: 10.1128/JVI.01542-10.
6. Liang W, Guan W, Chen R, Wang W, Li J, Xu K, Li C, Ai Q, Lu W, Liang H, Li S, He J. Cancer patients in SARS-CoV-2 infection: A nationwide analysis in China. *Lancet Oncol* 2020;21(3):335–337. doi: 10.1016/S1470-2045(20)30096-6.
7. Sidaway P. COVID-19 and cancer: What we know so far. *Nat Rev Clin Oncol* 2020;17(6):336. doi: 10.1038/s41571-020-0366-2.
8. Wang B, Huang Y. Which type of cancer patients are more susceptible to the SARS-COX-2: Evidence from a meta-analysis and bioinformatics analysis. *Crit Rev Oncol Hematol* 2020;153:103032. doi: 10.1016/j.critrevonc.2020.103032.
9. Aznab M. Evaluation of COVID 19 infection in 279 cancer patients treated during a 90-day period in 2020 pandemic. *Int J Clin Oncol* 2020;25(9):1581–1586. doi: 10.1007/s10147-020-01734-6.

10. ElGohary GM, Hashmi S, Styczynski J, Kharfan-Dabaja MA, Alblooshi RM, de la Cámara R, Mohmed S, Alshaibani A, Cesaro S, Abd El-Aziz N, Almaghrabi R, Gergis U, Majhail NS, El-Gohary Y, Chemaly RF, Aljurf M, El Fakih R. The risk and prognosis of COVID-19 infection in cancer patients: A systematic review and meta-analysis. *Hematol Oncol Stem Cell Ther* 2022;15(2):45–53. doi: 10.1016/j.hemonc.2020.07.005.

11. Zhang H, Quek K, Chen R, Chen J, Chen B. Expression of the SAR2-Cov-2 receptor ACE2 reveals the susceptibility of COVID-19 in non-small cell lung cancer. *J Cancer* 2020;11(18):5289–5292. doi: 10.7150/jca.49462.

12. Yang J, Li H, Hu S, Zhou Y. ACE2 correlated with immune infiltration serves as a prognostic biomarker in endometrial carcinoma and renal papillary cell carcinoma: Implication for COVID-19. *Aging* 2020;2(8):6518–6535. doi: 10.18632/aging.103100.

13. Ding S, Liang TJ. Is SARS-CoV-2 also an enteric pathogen with potential fecal-oral transmission? A COVID-19 virological and clinical review. *Gastroenterology* 2020 July;159(1):53–61. doi: 10.1053/j.gastro.2020.04.052.

14. Tan ND, Qiu Y, Xing XB, Ghosh S, Chen MH, Mao R. Associations between angiotensin-converting enzyme inhibitors and angiotensin II receptor blocker use, gastrointestinal symptoms, and mortality among patients with COVID-19. *Gastroenterology.* 2020;159(3):1170–1172. doi: 10.1053/j.gastro.2020.05.034.

15. Xu J, Chu M, Zhong F, Tan X, Tang G, Mai J, Lai N, Guan C, Liang Y, Liao G. Digestive symptoms of COVID-19 and expression of ACE2 in digestive tract organs. *Cell Death Discov* 2020;6:76. doi: 10.1038/s41420-020-00307-w.

16. Huang C, Wang Y, Li X, Ren L, Zhao J, Hu Y, Zhang L, Fan G, Xu J, Gu X, Cheng Z, Yu T, Xia J, Wei Y, Wu W, Xie X, Yin W, Li H, Liu M, Xiao Y, Gao H, Guo L, Xie J, Wang G, Jiang R, Gao Z, Jin Q, Wang J, Cao B. Clinical features of patients infected with 2019 novel coronavirus in Wuhan, China. *Lancet.* 2020;395(10223):497–506. doi: 10.1016/S0140-6736(20)30183-5.

17. Chen N, Zhou M, Dong X, Qu J, Gong F, Han Y, Qiu Y, Wang J, Liu Y, Wei Y, Xia J, Yu T, Zhang X, Zhang L. Epidemiological and clinical characteristics of 99 cases of 2019 novel coronavirus pneumonia in Wuhan, China: A descriptive study. *Lancet.* 2020;395(10223):507–513. doi: 10.1016/S0140-6736(20)30211-7.

18. Fang D, Ma JD, Guan J, Wang M, Yang Song Y, Tian D, Li P. Manifestations of digestive system in hospitalized patients with novel coronavirus pneumonia in Wuhan, China: A single-center, descriptive study, *Chin J Dig Dis* 2020;12:151–156. doi: 10.3760/cma.j.issn.0254-1432.2020.0005.

19. Wang D, Hu B, Hu C, Zhu F, Liu X, Zhang J, Wang B, Xiang H, Cheng Z, Xiong Y, Zhao Y, Li Y, Wang X, Peng Z. Clinical characteristics of 138 hospitalized patients with 2019 novel coronavirus-infected pneumonia in Wuhan, China. *JAMA* 2020 March;323(11):1061–1069. doi: 10.1001/jama.2020.1585.

20. Xiao F, Tang M, Zheng X, Liu Y, Li X, Shan H. Evidence for gastrointestinal infection of SARS-CoV-2. *Gastroenterology* 2020 May;158(6):1831–1833 doi: 10.1053/j. gastro.2020.02.055.

21. Xu XW, Wu XX, Jiang XG, Xu KJ, Ying LJ, Ma CL, Li SB, Wang HY, Zhang S, Gao HN, Sheng JF, Cai HL, Qiu YQ, Li LJ. Clinical findings in a group of patients infected with the 2019 novel coronavirus (SARS-Cov-2) outside of Wuhan, China: Retrospective case series. *BMJ* 2020;368:m606. doi: 10.1136/bmj.m606.

22. Lin L, Jiang X, Zhang Z, Huang S, Zhang Z, Fang Z, Gu Z, Gao L, Shi H, Mai L, Liu Y, Lin X, Lai R, Yan Z, Li X, Shan H. Gastrointestinal symptoms of 95 cases with SARS-CoV-2 infection. *Gut* 2020;69(6):997–1001. doi: 10.1136/gutjnl-2020-321013.

23. Sanz Segura P, Arguedas Lázaro Y, Mostacero Tapia S, Cabrera Chaves T, Sebastián Domingo JJ. Involvement of the digestive system in COVID-19. A review. *Gastroenterol Hepatol* 2020;43(8):464–471. doi: 10.1016/j.gastrohep.2020.06.004.

24. Wu F, Zhao S, Yu B, Chen YM, Wang W, Song ZG, Hu Y, Tao ZW, Tian JH, Pei YY, Yuan ML, Zhang YL, Dai FH, Liu Y, Wang QM, Zheng JJ, Xu L, Holmes EC, Zhang YZ. A new coronavirus associated with human respiratory disease in China. *Nature* 2020;579(7798):265–269. doi: 10.1038/s41586-020-2008-3.

25. Zhang H, Li HB, Lyu JR, Lei XM, Li W, Wu G, Lyu J, Dai ZM. Specific ACE2 expression in small intestinal enterocytes may cause gastrointestinal symptoms and injury after 2019-nCoV infection. *Int J Infect Dis* 2020;96:19–24. doi: 10.1016/j.ijid.2020.04.027.

26. Zhou J, Li C, Zhao G, Chu H, Wang D, Yan HH, Poon VK, Wen L, Wong BH, Zhao X, Chiu MC, Yang D, Wang Y, Au-Yeung RKH, Chan IH, Sun S, Chan JF, To KK, Memish ZA, Corman VM, Drosten C, Hung IF, Zhou Y, Leung SY, Yuen KY. Human intestinal tract serves as an alternative infection route for Middle East respiratory syndrome coronavirus. *Sci Adv* 2017 Nov 15;3(11):eaao4966. doi: 10.1126/sciadv.aao4966.

27. Jin X, Lian JS, Hu JH, Gao J, Zheng L, Zhang YM, Hao SR, Jia HY, Cai H, Zhang XL, Yu GD, Xu KJ, Wang XY, Gu JQ, Zhang SY, Ye CY, Jin CL, Lu YF, Yu X, Yu XP, Huang JR, Xu KL, Ni Q, Yu CB, Zhu B, Li YT, Liu J, Zhao H, Zhang X, Yu L, Guo YZ, Su JW, Tao JJ, Lang GJ, Wu XX, Wu WR, Qv TT, Xiang DR, Yi P, Shi D, Chen Y, Ren Y, Qiu YQ, Li LJ, Sheng J, Yang Y. Epidemiological, clinical and virological characteristics of 74 cases of coronavirus-infected disease 2019 (COVID-19) with gastrointestinal symptoms. *Gut* 2020;69(6):1002–1009. doi: 10.1136/gutjnl-2020-320926.

28. Sultan S, Altayar O, Siddique SM, Davitkov P, Feuerstein JD, Lim JK, Falck-Ytter Y, El-Serag HB, AGA Institute. Electronic address: ewilson@gastro.org. AGA Institute rapid review of the gastrointestinal and liver manifestations of COVID-19, meta-analysis of international data, and recommendations for the consultative management of patients with COVID-19. *Gastroenterology* 2020;159(1):320–334. doi: 10.1053/j.gastro.2020.05.001.

29. Zuo T, Zhang F, Lui GCY, Yeoh YK, Li AYL, Zhan H, Wan Y, Chung ACK, Cheung CP, Chen N, Lai CKC, Chen Z, Tso EYK, Fung KSC, Chan V, Ling L, Joynt G, Hui DSC, Chan FKL, Chan PKS, Ng SC. Alterations in gut microbiota of patients with COVID-19 during time of hospitalization. *Gastroenterology* 2020;159(3):944–955. doi: 10.1053/j.gastro.2020.05.048.

30. Yeoh YK, Zuo T, Lui GC, Zhang F, Liu Q, Li AY, Chung AC, Cheung CP, Tso EY, Fung KS, Chan V, Ling L, Joynt G, Hui DS, Chow KM, Ng SSS, Li TC, Ng RW, Yip TC, Wong GL, Chan FK, Wong CK, Chan PK, Ng SC. Gut microbiota composition reflects disease severity and dysfunctional immune responses in patients with COVID-19. *Gut* 2021;70(4):698–706. doi: 10.1136/gutjnl-2020-323020.

31. Gu S, Chen Y, Wu Z, Chen Y, Gao H, Lv L, Guo F, Zhang X, Luo R, Huang C, Lu H, Zheng B, Zhang J, Yan R, Zhang H, Jiang H, Xu Q, Guo J, Gong Y, Tang L, Li L. Alterations of the gut microbiota in patients with coronavirus disease 2019 or H1N1 influenza. *Clin Infect Dis* 2020;71(10):2669–2678. doi: 10.1093/cid/ciaa709.

32. Nori P, Cowman K, Chen V, Bartash R, Szymczak W, Madaline T, Punjabi Katiyar C, Jain R, Aldrich M, Weston G, Gialanella P, Corpuz M, Gendlina I, Guo Y. Bacterial and fungal coinfections in COVID-19 patients hospitalized during the New York City pandemic surge. *Infect Control Hosp Epidemiol* 2021;42(1):84–88. doi: 10.1017/ice.2020.368.

33. Grasselli G, Scaravilli V, Mangioni D, Scudeller L, Alagna L, Bartoletti M, Bellani G, Biagioni E, Bonfanti P, Bottino N, Coloretti I, Cutuli SL, De Pascale G, Ferlicca D, Fior G, Forastieri A, Franzetti M, Greco M, Guzzardella A, Linguadoca S, Meschiari M, Messina A, Monti G, Morelli P, Muscatello A, Redaelli S, Stefanini F, Tonetti T, Antonelli M, Cecconi M, Foti G, Fumagalli R, Girardis M, Ranieri M, Viale P, Raviglione M, Pesenti A, Gori A, Bandera A. Hospital-acquired infections in critically ill patients with COVID-19. *Chest* 2021;160(2):454–465. doi: 10.1016/j. chest.2021.04.002.

34. Yu D, Ininbergs K, Hedman K, Giske CG, Strålin K, Özenci V. Low prevalence of bloodstream infection and high blood culture contamination rates in patients with COVID-19. *PLOS ONE* 2020;15(11):e0242533. doi: 10.1371/journal.pone.0242533.

35. Langford BJ, So M, Raybardhan S, Leung V, Westwood D, MacFadden DR, Soucy JR, Daneman N. Bacterial co-infection and secondary infection in patients with COVID-19: A living rapid review and meta-analysis. *Clin Microbiol Infect* 2020;26(12):1622–1629. doi: 10.1016/j.cmi.2020.07.016.

36. Shafran N, Shafran I, Ben-Zvi H, Sofer S, Sheena L, Krause I, Shlomai A, Goldberg E, Sklan EH. Secondary bacterial infection in COVID-19 patients is a stronger predictor for death compared to influenza patients. *Sci Rep* 2021;11(1):12703. doi: 10.1038/s41598-021-92220-0.

37. Wu D, Ding Y, Wang T, Cui P, Huang L, Min Z, Xu M. Significance of tumor-infiltrating immune cells in the prognosis of colon cancer. *Onco Targets Ther* 2020;22(13):4581–4589. doi: 10.2147/OTT.S250416.

38. Yang L, Chai P, Yu J, Fan X. Effects of cancer on patients with COVID-19: A systematic review and meta-analysis of 63,019 participants. *Cancer Biol Med* 2021 15;18(1):298–307. doi: 10.20892/j.issn.2095-3941.2020.0559.

39. He X, Lau EHY, Wu P, Deng X, Wang J, Hao X, Lau YC, Wong JY, Guan Y, Tan X, Mo X, Chen Y, Liao B, Chen W, Hu F, Zhang Q, Zhong M, Wu Y, Zhao L, Zhang F, Cowling BJ, Li F, Leung GM. Temporal dynamics in viral shedding and transmissibility of COVID-19. *Nat Med.* 2020;26(5):672–675. doi: 10.1038/s41591-020-0869-5.

40. Xu K, Cai H, Shen Y, Ni Q, Chen Y, Hu S, Li J, Wang H, Yu L, Huang H, Qiu Y, Wei G, Fang Q, Zhou J, Sheng J, Liang T, Li L. Management of COVID-19: The Zhejiang experience. *Zhejiang Da Xue Xue Bao Yi Xue Ban.* 2020;49(2):147–157. doi: 10.3785/j.issn.1008-9292.2020.02.02.

41. Hashimoto T, Perlot T, Rehman A, Trichereau J, Ishiguro H, Paolino M, Sigl V, Hanada T, Hanada R, Lipinski S, Wild B, Camargo SM, Singer D, Richter A, Kuba K, Fukamizu A, Schreiber S, Clevers H, Verrey F, Rosenstiel P, Penninger JM. ACE2 links amino acid malnutrition to microbial ecology and intestinal inflammation. *Nature* 2012;487(7408):477–481. doi: 10.1038/nature11228.

42. Wu C, Chen X, Cai Y, Xia J, Zhou X, Xu S, Huang H, Zhang L, Zhou X, Du C, Zhang Y, Song J, Wang S, Chao Y, Yang Z, Xu J, Zhou X, Chen D, Xiong W, Xu L, Zhou F, Jiang J, Bai C, Zheng J, Song Y. Risk factors associated with acute respiratory distress syndrome and death in patients with coronavirus disease 2019 pneumonia in Wuhan, China. *JAMA Intern Med* 2020;180(7):934–943. doi: 10.1001/jamainternmed.2020.0994.

43. Neurath MF. COVID-19 and immunomodulation in IBD. *Gut* 2020;69(7):1335–1342. doi: 10.1136/gutjnl-2020-321269.

44. Zhang M, Zhou Q, Dorfman RG, Huang X, Fan T, Zhang H, Zhang J, Yu C. Butyrate inhibits interleukin-17 and generates Tregs to ameliorate colorectal colitis in rats. *BMC Gastroenterol* 2016;16(1):84. doi: 10.1186/s12876-016-0500-x.

45. Niu M, Chen P. Crosstalk between gut microbiota and sepsis. *Burns Trauma* 2021;9:tkab036. doi: 10.1093/burnst/tkab036.
46. Qian Q, Fan L, Liu W, Li J, Yue J, Wang M, Ke X, Yin Y, Chen Q, Jiang C. Direct evidence of active SARS-CoV-2 replication in the intestine. *Clin Infect Dis* 2021 2;73(3):361–366. doi: 10.1093/cid/ciaa925.
47. Kumar A, Faiq MA, Pareek V, Raza K, Narayan RK, Prasoon P, Kumar P, Kulandhasamy M, Kumari C, Kant K, Singh HN, Qadri R, Pandey SN, Kumar S. Relevance of SARS-CoV-2 related factors ACE2 and TMPRSS2 expressions in gastrointestinal tissue with pathogenesis of digestive symptoms, diabetes-associated mortality, and disease recurrence in COVID-19 patients. *Med Hypotheses* 2020;144:110271. doi: 10.1016/j.mehy.2020.110271.
48. Shafiee S, Cegolon L, Khafaei M, Gholami N, Zhao S, Khalesi N, Moosavian H, Fathi S, Izadi M, Ghadian A, Javanbakht M, Javanbakht A, Akhavan-Sigari R. Gastrointestinal cancers, ACE-2/TMPRSS2 expression and susceptibility to COVID-19. *Cancer Cell Int* 2021 16;21(1):431. doi: 10.1186/s12935-021-02129-x.
49. Bernardi S, Zennaro C, Palmisano S, Velkoska E, Sabato N, Toffoli B, Giacomel G, Buri L, Zanconati F, Bellini G, Burrell LM, De Manzini N, Fabris B. Characterization and significance of ACE2 and Mas receptor in human colon adenocarcinoma. *J Renin Angiotensin Aldosterone Syst* 2012;13(1):202–209. doi: 10.1177/1470320311426023.
50. Chen Y, Gong W, Wei H, Dai W, Xu S. 2019-nCoV may create complications in colon cancer patients with ACE2 expression. *Int J Clin Exp Pathol* 2020;13(9):2305–2311.
51. Darvish-Damavandi M, Laycock J, Ward C, van Driel MS, Goldgraben MA, Buczacki SJ. An analysis of SARS-CoV-2 cell entry genes identifies the intestine and colorectal cancer as susceptible tissues. *Br J Surg* 2020;107(11):e452–e454. doi: 10.1002/bjs.11911.
52. Liu C, Wang K, Zhang M, Hu X, Hu T, Liu Y, Hu Q, Wu S, Yue J. High expression of ACE2 and TMPRSS2 and clinical characteristics of COVID-19 in colorectal cancer patients. *NPJ Precis Oncol* 2021;5(1):1. doi: 10.1038/s41698-020-00139-y.
53. Wang H, Yang J. Colorectal cancer that highly express both ACE2 and TMPRSS2, suggesting severe symptoms to SARS-CoV-2 infection. *Pathol Oncol Res* 2021;27:612969. doi: 10.3389/pore.2021.612969.
54. Ahmadi M, Pashangzadeh S, Mousavi P, Saffarzadeh N, Amin Habibi M, Hajiesmaeili F, Rezaei N. ACE2 correlates with immune infiltrates in colon adenocarcinoma: Implication for COVID-19. *Int Immunopharmacol* 2021;95:107568. doi: 10.1016/j.intimp.2021.107568.
55. Francescangeli F, De Angelis ML, Zeuner A. COVID-19: A potential driver of immune-mediated breast cancer recurrence? *Breast Cancer Res* 2020;22(1):117. doi: 10.1186/s13058-020-01360-0.
56. Albrengues J, Shields MA, Ng D, Park CG, Ambrico A, Poindexter ME, Upadhyay P, Uyeminami DL, Pommier A, Küttner V, Bružas E, Maiorino L, Bautista C, Carmona EM, Gimotty PA, Fearon DT, Chang K, Lyons SK, Pinkerton KE, Trotman LC, Goldberg MS, Yeh JT, Egeblad M. Neutrophil extracellular traps produced during inflammation awaken dormant cancer cells in mice. *Science* 2018;361(6409):eaao4227. doi: 10.1126/science.aao4227.
57. Fluegen G, Avivar-Valderas A, Wang Y, Padgen MR, Williams JK, Nobre AR, Calvo V, Cheung JF, Bravo-Cordero JJ, Entenberg D, Castracane J, Verkhusha V, Keely PJ, Condeelis J, Aguirre-Ghiso JA. Phenotypic heterogeneity of disseminated tumour cells is preset by primary tumour hypoxic microenvironments. *Nat Cell Biol* 2017;19(2):120–132. doi: 10.1038/ncb3465.

58. Barbieri A, Robinson N, Palma G, Maurea N, Desiderio V, Botti G. Can beta-2-adrenergic pathway be a new target to combat SARS-CoV-2 hyperinflammatory syndrome?-lessons learned from cancer. *Front Immunol* 2020;11:588724. doi: 10.3389/fimmu.2020.588724.

59. Zhang Q, Lu S, Li T, Yu L, Zhang Y, Zeng H, Qian X, Bi J, Lin Y. ACE2 inhibits breast cancer angiogenesis via suppressing the VEGFa/VEGFR2/ERK pathway. *J Exp Clin Cancer Res* 2019;38(1):173. doi: 10.1186/s13046-019-1156-5.

60. Qian YR, Guo Y, Wan HY, Fan L, Feng Y, Ni L, Xiang Y, Li QY. Angiotensin-converting enzyme 2 attenuates the metastasis of non-small cell lung cancer through inhibition of epithelial-mesenchymal transition. *Oncol Rep* 2013;29(6):2408–2414. doi: 10.3892/or.2013.2370.

61. Yu C, Tang W, Wang Y, Shen Q, Wang B, Cai C, Meng X, Zou F. Downregulation of ACE2/Ang-(1–7)/Mas axis promotes breast cancer metastasis by enhancing store-operated calcium entry. *Cancer Lett* 2016;376(2):268–277. doi: 10.1016/j.canlet.2016.04.006.

62. Li J, Yang ZL, Ren X, Zou Q, Yuan Y, Liang L, Chen M, Chen S. ACE2 and FZD1 are prognosis markers in squamous cell/adenosquamous carcinoma and adenocarcinoma of gallbladder. *J Mol Histol* 2014;45(1):47–57. doi: 10.1007/s10735-013-9528-1.

63. Zhong W, Li J, Kong M, Gao Q, Teng X, Liang T, Zhang J. The encounter of tumor and SARS-CoV-2: Pathological findings in a patient with colon cancer and COVID-19 Preprint from Research Square, 01 July 2020. DOI: 10.21203/rs.3.rs-38812/v1 PPR: PPR182504.

64. Ottaiano A, Scala S, D'Alterio C, Trotta A, Bello A, Rea G, Picone C, Santorsola M, Petrillo A, Nasti G. Unexpected tumor reduction in metastatic colorectal cancer patients during SARS-Cov-2 infection. *Ther Adv Med Oncol* 2021;13:17588359211011455. doi: 10.1177/17588359211011455.

65. Ottaiano A, Santorsola M, Circelli L, Cascella M, Petrillo N, Perri F, Casillo M, Granata V, Ianniello M, Izzo F, Picone C, Correra M, Petrillo A, Sirica R, Misso G, Delrio P, Nasti G, Savarese G, Caraglia M. Genetic landscape of colorectal cancer patients manifesting tumor shrinkage during SARS-Cov-2 infection. *Ther Adv Med Oncol* 2022;8(14):17588359221138388. doi: 10.1177/17588359221138388.

66. Chen H, Zhang F, Zhang J, Zhang X, Guo Y, Yao Q. A holistic view of berberine inhibiting intestinal carcinogenesis in conventional mice based on microbiome-metabolomics analysis. *Front Immunol* 2020;11:588079. doi: 10.3389/fimmu.2020.588079.

67. Gill SR, Pop M, Deboy RT, Eckburg PB, Turnbaugh PJ, Samuel BS, Gordon JI, Relman DA, Fraser-Liggett CM, Nelson KE. Metagenomic analysis of the human distal gut microbiome. *Science* 2006;312(5778):1355–1359. doi: 10.1126/science.1124234.

68. Howell MC, Green R, McGill AR, Dutta R, Mohapatra S, Mohapatra SS. SARS-CoV-2-induced gut microbiome dysbiosis: Implications for colorectal cancer. *Cancers* 2021;13(11):2676. doi: 10.3390/cancers13112676.

69. Bao R, Hernandez K, Huang L, Luke JJ. ACE2 and TMPRSS2 expression by clinical, HLA, immune, and microbial correlates across 34 human cancers and matched normal tissues: Implications for SARS-CoV-2 COVID-19. *J Immunother Cancer* 2020;8(2):e001020. doi: 10.1136/jitc-2020-001020.

70. Lamers MM, Beumer J, van der Vaart J, Knoops K, Puschhof J, Breugem TI, Ravelli RBG, Paul van Schayck J, Mykytyn AZ, Duimel HQ, van Donselaar E, Riesebosch S, Kuijpers HJH, Schipper D, van de Wetering WJ, de Graaf M, Koopmans M, Cuppen E, Peters PJ, Haagmans BL, Clevers H. SARS-CoV-2 productively infects human gut enterocytes. *Science* 2020 Jul 3;369(6499):50–54. doi: 10.1126/science.abc1669.

71. Zang R, Gomez Castro MF, McCune BT, Zeng Q, Rothlauf PW, Sonnek NM, Liu Z, Brulois KF, Wang X, Greenberg HB, Diamond MS, Ciorba MA, Whelan SPJ, Ding S. TMPRSS2 and TMPRSS4 promote SARS-CoV-2 infection of human small intestinal enterocytes. *Sci Immunol* 2020;5(47):eabc3582. doi: 10.1126/sciimmunol. abc3582.

72. Sánchez-Alcoholado L, Ramos-Molina B, Otero A, Laborda-Illanes A, Ordóñez R, Medina JA, Gómez-Millán J, Queipo-Ortuño MI. The role of the gut microbiome in colorectal cancer development and therapy response. *Cancers* 2020 29;12(6):1406. doi: 10.3390/cancers12061406.

73. Ma WT, Yao XT, Peng Q, Chen DK. The protective and pathogenic roles of IL-17 in viral infections: Friend or foe? *Open Biol* 2019 26;9(7):190109. doi: 10.1098/rsob.190109.

74. Gu S, Chen Y, Wu Z, Chen Y, Gao H, Lv L, Guo F, Zhang X, Luo R, Huang C, Lu H, Zheng B, Zhang J, Yan R, Zhang H, Jiang H, Xu Q, Guo J, Gong Y, Tang L, Li L. Alterations of the gut microbiota in patients with coronavirus disease 2019 or H1N1 influenza. *Clin Infect Dis* 2020;71(10):2669–2678. doi: 10.1093/cid/ciaa709.

75. Tao W, Zhang G, Wang X, Guo M, Zeng W, Xu Z, Cao D, Pan A, Wang Y, Zhang K, Ma X, Chen Z, Jin T, Liu L, Weng J, Zhu S. Analysis of the intestinal microbiota in COVID-19 patients and its correlation with the inflammatory factor IL-18. *Med Microecol* 2020;5:100023. doi: 10.1016/j.medmic.2020.100023.

76. Zhang H, Ai JW, Yang W, Zhou X, He F, Xie S, Zeng W, Li Y, Yu Y, Gou X, Li Y, Wang X, Su H, Zhu Z, Xu T, Zhang W. Metatranscriptomic characterization of coronavirus disease 2019 identified a host transcriptional classifier associated with immune signaling. *Clin Infect Dis* 2021;73(3):376–385. doi: 10.1093/cid/ciaa663.

77. Tang L, Gu S, Gong Y, Li B, Lu H, Li Q, Zhang R, Gao X, Wu Z, Zhang J, Zhang Y, Li L. Clinical significance of the correlation between changes in the major intestinal bacteria species and COVID-19 severity. *Engineering* 2020;6(10):1178–1184. doi: 10.1016/j.eng.2020.05.013.

78. Zuo T, Liu Q, Zhang F, Lui GC, Tso EY, Yeoh YK, Chen Z, Boon SS, Chan FK, Chan PK, Ng SC. Depicting SARS-CoV-2 faecal viral activity in association with gut microbiota composition in patients with COVID-19. *Gut* 2021;70(2):276–284. doi: 10.1136/gutjnl-2020-322294.

79. Zuo T, Zhan H, Zhang F, Liu Q, Tso EYK, Lui GCY, Chen N, Li A, Lu W, Chan FKL, Chan PKS, Ng SC. Alterations in fecal fungal microbiome of patients with COVID-19 during time of hospitalization until discharge. *Gastroenterology* 2020 Oct;159(4):1302–1310. doi: 10.1053/j.gastro.2020.06.048.

80. Jayasimhan A, Mariño E. Dietary SCFAs, IL-22, and GFAP: The three musketeers in the gut-neuro-immune network in type 1 diabetes. *Front Immunol* 2019;10:2429. doi: 10.3389/fimmu.2019.02429.

81. McNabney SM, Henagan TM. Short chain fatty acids in the colon and peripheral tissues: A focus on butyrate, colon cancer, obesity and insulin resistance. *Nutrients* 2017;9(12):1348. doi: 10.3390/nu9121348.

82. Sun CH, Li BB, Wang B, Zhao J, Zhang XY, Li TT, Li WB, Tang D, Qiu MJ, Wang XC, Zhu CM, Qian ZR. The role of *Fusobacterium nucleatum* in colorectal cancer: From carcinogenesis to clinical management. *Chronic Dis Transl Med* 2019;5(3):178–187. doi: 10.1016/j.cdtm.2019.09.001.

83. Amenta EM, Spallone A, Rodriguez-Barradas MC, El Sahly HM, Atmar RL, Kulkarni PA. Postacute COVID-19: An overview and approach to classification. *Open Forum Infect Dis* 2020;7(12):ofaa509. doi: 10.1093/ofid/ofaa509.

84. Carfì A, Bernabei R, Landi F. Gemelli against COVID-19 post-acute care study group. Persistent symptoms in patients after acute COVID-19. *JAMA* 2020;324(6):603–605. doi: 10.1001/jama.2020.12603.
85. Howell MC, Green R, McGill AR, Dutta R, Mohapatra S, Mohapatra SS. SARS-CoV-2-induced gut microbiome dysbiosis: Implications for colorectal cancer. *Cancers* 2021;13(11):2676. doi: 10.3390/cancers13112676.
86. Cai C, Zhang X, Liu Y, Shen E, Feng Z, Guo C, Han Y, Ouyang Y, Shen H. Gut microbiota imbalance in colorectal cancer patients, the risk factor of COVID-19 mortality. *Gut Pathog* 2021;13(1):70. doi: 10.1186/s13099-021-00466-w.

9

Viral Shedding and Long COVID-19 Disease in Cancer Patients

Gabriella Marfe, Stefania Perna, Giovanna Mirone, and Arvind Kumar Shukla

Introduction

In December 2019, beta-coronavirus was identified and named as severe acute respiratory syndrome coronavirus 2 (SARS-CoV-2). This virus has caused a pandemic called coronavirus disease 2019 (COVID-19), with a very high number of cases and deaths globally [1, 2]. This pandemic represented a grim and complex situation and significant challenge to governments worldwide due to the transmissibility of the virus, the scale of its impact on morbidity and mortality, the uncertainty regarding the development of long-term immunity in those infected, and the impact on health-care systems, economies, and society [3, 4]. During the pandemic, different studies have reported that cancer patients were vulnerable to the severe symptoms of the viral disease. One study was carried out on a sample of 536 non-cancer patients and 105 cancer patients of the same age and infected with COVID-19. The authors found that the cancer patients had more severe disease when compared with patients without cancer. Furthermore, patients with metastatic cancer and positive COVID-19 had a higher death risk [5]. In another study, the author found that 18 cancer patients sample out of 1590 COVID-19 positive cases had more severe disease than no cancer patients [6]. Desai et al observed that SARS-CoV-2–infected cancer patients after a surgery or chemotherapy had high risk for a severe complication [7]. In another study, Zhang et al showed that 53.6% of COVID-19–infected cancer patients developed severe COVID symptoms and 28.6% of patients died [8]. In another study, the authors found a high mortality rate in patients suffering from lung (55%), gastrointestinal (upper-GI) (38%), pancreatic (67%), colorectal (38%), and gynecological (38%) cancers [9]. Furthermore, in a recent study, the authors have reported that 229 cancer patients (14.96%) of 1,524,228 (14.96%) had non-small cell lung cancer (NSCLC). These patients, older than 60 years of age (4.3%), were found to be more vulnerable to COVID-19 than those aged 60 years or less (1.8%) [10]. Another study found that patients with oral cancer (stage IV)–treated anti-cancer therapy and infected with COVID-19 had severe symptoms and an increased death rate when compared with those patients who did not contract COVID-19 after the anti-cancer treatments [11]. Hence, it is imperative to understand why cancer patients are so prone to this deadly viral disease. In the present chapter, we try to understand the association among the prolonged viral shedding clinical symptoms and long COVID-19 in these patients after or during their therapy.

DOI: 10.1201/9781003362562-10

Viral Shedding in Cancer Patients

The RNA of this virus can be identified in several sites of the human body such as nares, nasopharynx, pharynx, bronchoalveolar lavage (BAL) fluid, feces, and blood [12–14]. SARS-CoV-2 RNA shedding can last from 3 until 46 days after symptom onset [15–17]. Furthermore, many studies reported that there is no difference regarding duration and viral load between symptomatic and asymptomatic individuals [18–20]. Persistent SARS-CoV-2 RNA shedding has been documented, with patients remaining qRT-PCR-positive (real-time quantitative reverse transcription PCR) for up to 63 days [21, 22]. In addition, there were reports of symptomatic and asymptomatic individuals testing positive again after a period of negative testing [23, 24]. Moreover, many studies estimated that infectiousness began 2.3 days prior to symptom onset and declined within 7 days of symptom onset [25]. In this regard, it was possible to isolate from patients' samples the infectious SARS-CoV-2 up to 8 days after symptom onset but typically not thereafter [26, 27]. In contrast to prolonged shedding of SARS-CoV-2 RNA, the longest detected shedding of infectious SARS-CoV-2 virus was up to 20 days after the initial positive test result [22, 28]. The probability of isolating SARS-CoV-2 decreased with a lower viral load, when the duration of symptoms exceeded 15 days, and upon generation of detectable neutralising antibodies [28]. Viral shedding in stool samples is prolonged and sometimes erratic. Many studies reported no evidence of successful virus isolation from stool samples. In a study published on 18 May 2020, the authors were able to isolate SARS-CoV-2 virus from stool samples in two of the three patients tested [29]. Furthermore, Parasa et al found that SARS-CoV-2 RNA was detected in the stool samples of 41% of patients, and that 12% of all COVID-19 patients reported gastrointestinal symptoms [30]. The relationship between SARS-CoV-2 detection, viral load, and infectivity is not fully understood, as the presence of viral RNA may not represent transmissible live virus. Moreover, some studies reported that COVID-19 patients are infectious from one to three days before symptom onset, although viable virus has been successfully isolated from upper respiratory tract samples up to six days before onset of symptoms [31]. Two separate epidemiological investigations concluded that there was high transmissibility near, and even before symptom onset [32, 33]. Furthermore, no statistically significant difference in the viral load between symptomatic and asymptomatic patient samples was found in two included studies [34, 35]. A secondary analysis of published data by Casey et al estimated the proportion of pre-symptomatic transmission to be approximately 56% [36]. Furthermore, in two different studies, the authors did not detect infectious isolates from any sample after eight days from symptom onset in spite of ongoing high viral loads [37, 38]. However, the duration of infectivity remains uncertain as two recent studies have reported isolation of viable virus from upper and lower respiratory samples 13 days (maximum follow-up) and 18 days respectively after symptom onset.

What about cancer patients? In these patients the situation is very complicated because the infectivity can lead to isolation and other precautionary activities delaying therapy, tests, and other procedures. But, in most cases, recurrent or prolonged test positivity does not necessarily mean infectiousness. In this regard, the interruption of crucial chemotherapy for any prolonged duration of time can be highly inappropriate, and the risk–benefit ratio would definitely be favorable towards continuation of chemotherapy, even if the patient is found to be positive. At the beginning of the pandemic, the American Society of Clinical Oncology (ASCO) recommended that all cancer patients with a diagnosis of COVID-19 should cease cancer directed therapy (CDT) for risk assessment [39]. The guidelines recommend a pause in CDT administration for 14 days for a majority of patients and/or until symptom free for 72 hours including a negative test on two consecutive nasopharyngeal (NP) polymerase chain reaction (PCR) swabs, which are at least 24 hours apart. Different studies reported conflicting results whether CDTs actually increase COVID-19 related morbidity and mortality [40]. Outcomes are likely dependent on tumour histology, type of CDT, and severity of COVID-19 symptoms. A retrospective analysis was carried out with 299 cancer patients undergoing cancer-directed therapy (CDT) and tested for SARS-CoV-2 using nasopharyngeal nested PCR assay at Columbia University Medical Irving Medical Center (CUIMC). Among them 77 tested positive and the authors analysed 26 positive cancer patients with mild-to-moderate COVID-19 receiving CDT. The nested PCR test was repeated every 1 to 2 weeks until two successive negatives. Twenty patients had sequential negative swabs after 14 days and therapy was delayed in 21 patients of whom three experienced disease progression, likely attributed to an interruption in CDT, which was delayed by a mean of 53 days. Furthermore, 16 patients in CDT were positive for IgG antibodies at the time of consent, despite protracted viral detectability by nested PCR. In summary, the authors observed that the cancer patients receiving CDT appeared to have prolonged detectable viral positivity by PCR. In this regard, the authors recommend that patients having from asymptomatic to mild COVID-19 but with aggressive malignancies were at greatest risk for cancer-related morbidity and mortality due to CDT cessation and should be considered for continued CDT without interruption [41]. Other studies defined a high risk for severe COVID-19 patients with past or active malignancy and patients that are post-cytotoxic chemotherapy [42–44]. In these patients, immune response can be limited by the chronic immunosuppressed state, which causes reduced plasmacytoid dendritic cells available to respond to infection [45–46]. Furthermore, these patients are subject to lower levels of adaptive immunity and antibody production in the context of SARS-CoV-2 infection [47, 48]. This phenotype is correlated with lymphopenias, neutropenia, and decreased types I and III IFN response [49, 50]. These data provide framework for understanding how immune responses can be aberrantly affected in patients with cancer depending on the viral variant, host factors, type of underlying malignancy, and the impact of certain chemotherapeutic regimens on immunologic axes. Recent studies have described some of the mechanisms behind the blunted immune response in patients with cancer [51]. In another study, patients with hematologic malignancies hospitalised with COVID-19 had worse COVID-19 outcomes due to depletion of CD4+ and CD8+ T cells or lower B cell immunity [52]. In this regard, patients with hematologic malignancy who recovered from COVID-19 displayed lingering immunological consequences with impaired adaptive lymphocytic and innate myelomonocytic parameter [53]. For example, a case report showed a COVID-19 case with prolonged viral shedding for 2 months since the cell-mediated immunity of the patient was depressed (CD4+T cell <100/µl) following advanced malignant lymphoma and chemotherapy which had been completed 4 months prior to the onset of COVID-19 symptoms. The patient was treated with several treatments against COVID-19, however the results of polymerase chain reaction (PCR) from nasopharyngeal specimens remained positive for SARS-CoV-2 for 2 months. After 69 days, the patient tested negative with two consecutive PCR tests for SARS-CoV-2 [54]. In this scenario, an important consequence of this blunted immune response is prolonged viral clearance in patients with cancer, which can result in prolonged illness [55]. One study analysed the nasopharyngeal swabs from over 1,000 patients with and without cancer to compare duration of viral shedding of SARS-CoV-2 by RT-PCR–based cycle threshold (C_t) values and determined that an active malignancy conferred a longer shedding period associated with sustained presence of type 1 IFN [56]. Furthermore, in another study of 20 immunocompromised patients with COVID-19, viable virus could be isolated for up to 63 days post-symptom onset, while viral RNA was detectable for up to 78 days [57]. In clinical practice, prolonged viral shedding, even if the viral particles are no longer viable, usually precludes continuation of cancer therapy, with potential deleterious outcome of cancer progression [45]. Many studies confirmed that haematological malignancies (HM) patients have more severe and prolonged COVID-19 than patients with solid malignancies (SM) or patients treated with immunomodulatory medications for non-malignant diseases. A recent retrospective analysis examined the clinical presentation and outcome of 98,951 patients with COVID-19 in Catalonia, Spain [58]. The clinical and epidemiological data indicated that HM patients infected with COVID-19 have protracted viral shedding and possibly longer infectivity than SM patients [58]. Many research articles reported an association between polymerase chain reaction (PCR) cycle threshold (C_t) and infectivity [59, 60]. For instance, HM patients had generally the highest risk of prolonged shedding, as evidenced by nasal swabs with $C_t > 30$. In one study, PCR tests remained positive for a mean of 21.2 days in HM patients compared to 7.4 in matched controls without HM [61]. Serological studies indicated a similar pattern, with nasopharyngeal shedding and seroconversion both taking twice as long in HM patients (HR 1.97, 95% CI [1.56–2.38]) [62]. These differences seem to be larger among patients treated with anti-CD20, CAR T cell, or HCT recipients [63–64]. A case report published in *Cell* described a female patient with chronic lymphocytic leukemia and acquired hypogammaglobulinemia (a condition characterised by low levels of immunoglobulins, or antibodies) who had asymptomatic COVID-19. This patient shed infectious SARS-CoV-2 up to 70 days after her COVID-19 diagnosis, and genomic and subgenomic viral RNA could be isolated up to 105 days after diagnosis [65]. In another case report the authors described a 50-year-old male patient with splenic marginal zone lymphoma, with splenic and bone marrow involvement. After 6 cycles of chemo-immunotherapy (rituximab plus adriamcyin, cyclophosphamide, vincristine, and methylprednisolone), the patient achieved remission. After 1 year with pancytopenia with splenic and bone marrow involvement, partial remission was achieved with second-line chemo-immunotherapy with 6 cycles of rituximab and bendamustine. In the last months of 2019, a second relapse was observed and third-line chemo-immunotherapy with rituximab-phosphamide carboplatin and etoposide were commenced. After the completion of the second cycle, the patient was hospitalised with febrile neutropenia and pneumonia in January 2020. The patient tested PCR positive for 110 days in total; PCR positive for 60 consecutive days and tested positive after testing negative 2 times [66]. Another study reported the 21-plus days isolation of severe acute respiratory syndrome coronavirus 2 (SARS-CoV-2) in seven patients with a diagnosis of acute leukemia and confirmation of coronavirus disease (COVID-19) admitted to the Haematology Department of the Guillermo Almenara Irigoyen National Hospital (Lima, Peru) between October 2020 and February 2021, in which none of the subjects developed severe or critical sickness. The diagnosis was made from an antigenic test or reverse transcriptase polymerase chain reaction (RTPCR), which were taken through a nasopharyngeal swab that was performed as a prerequisite to the initiation of specific treatment for the underlying disease. Most of them were adults and had a diagnosis of acute lymphoblastic leukemia in remission and were awaiting their next course of chemotherapy. Viral RNA was isolated for more than 82 days after initial diagnosis (from 21 to 82 days). The case with the longest positive test time was for a patient with disease relapse, who developed a moderate type of COVID-19. At the date of the report, six patients were alive and one died due to the haematological disease activity [67]. In another case study, the authors found that patients with B-cell lymphomas were at particularly high risk for persistent SARS-CoV-2 positivity. Further analysis of these patients identified discrete risk factors for initial disease severity as compared to disease chronicity. Active therapy and diminished T-cell counts were drivers of acute mortality in COVID-19–infected patients with lymphoma. Conversely, B-cell-depleting therapy was the primary driver of re-hospitalisation for COVID-19. Furthermore, in the patients with persistent SARS-CoV-2 positivity, the authors observed high levels of viral entropy. These results suggested that persistent COVID-19 infection could be likely to remain a risk in patients with impaired adaptive immunity and that additional therapeutic strategies are needed to enable viral clearance in this high-risk population [68]. Martínez-Barranco and colleagues examined five patients with a follicular lymphoma (FL), who developed several episodes of COVID-19 after treatment with immunochemotherapy. All patients required hospitalisation due to pneumonia with severity criteria and were re-admitted after a median of 22 days [13–41] from the previous discharge. Furthermore, all showed B cell depletion by immunophenotyping, and no traces of immunoglobulin antibodies against SARS-CoV-2 [69]. Another study reported the case of a 71-year-old man with COVID-19 and mantle cell lymphoma, and rituximab-associated immunodeficiency. The clinical course was severe, unremitting, and prolonged, and viral shedding and failure to develop anti-severe acute respiratory syndrome coronavirus 2 antibodies continued for at least 6 months [70]. In another study, Santarelli et al described the clinical course of three patients with haematological neoplasms who contracted COVID-19 and they were not vaccinated. The first patient, a 22-year-old male with a refractory acute lymphoblastic leukaemia reported an oligosymptomatic COVID-19 with C_t of 23 with an ascending curve. The second patient, another male, aged 23, with a promyelocytic leukaemia, had recently begun treatment. He had a severe course with high oxygen requirements. His Ct decrease from 28, when he had fever, until to 14.8, during the ventilatory support. Viral clearance was documented 126 days after the beginning of the symptoms. Finally, a 60-year-old male had received rituximab as maintenance therapy for a follicular lymphoma 3 months before contracting COVID-19. He had a fulminant course and required mechanical ventilation a few days later. We highlight the association between the course of COVID-19 and the C_t. Viral shedding was longer than in immunocompetent hosts [71]. Retrospective case series were carried out as a single-centre analysis of 41 patients with haematological malignancies who developed COVID-19 between 8 March and 8 April 2020, at University Hospital Infanta Leonor, Madrid. Among these patients, 38 tested positive for RT-PCT, while the remaining three patients, who tested PCR negative, were diagnosed with COVID-19 on clinical grounds [72]. In another case report, a patient with follicular lymphoma and treated with an anti-CD20 antibody (obinutuzumab) was infected by COVID-19. This patient had persistent RT-PCR positivity and live virus isolation for 9 months despite treatment with remdesivir and other potential antiviral therapies. Furthermore, viral pneumonia repeatedly appeared and disappeared in different lobes as shown by the computed tomography image of the chest as if a new infection had occurred continuously. His SARS-CoV-2 antibody titer was negative during the illness, even after two doses of the BNT162b2 mRNA vaccine were administered in the seventh month of infection. A combination of monoclonal antibody therapy against COVID-19 (casirivimab and imdevimab) and antivirals resulted in negative RT-PCR results, and the virus was no longer isolated. During the 9-month active infection period, mutations were not evident in spike (S) protein were not detected mutations, and the in vitro susceptibility to remdesivir was retained. Therapeutic administration of anti-SARS-CoV-2 monoclonal antibodies is essential in immunocompromised patients [73]. Another study measured SARS-CoV-2 viral load using cycle threshold (CT) values from reverse-transcription polymerase chain reaction assays applied to nasopharyngeal swab specimens in 100 patients with cancer and 2,914 without cancer who were admitted to three New York City hospitals. Overall, the in-hospital mortality rate was 38.8% among patients with a high viral load, 24.1% among patients with a medium viral load, and 15.3% among patients with a low viral load ($p < 0.001$). Similar findings were observed in patients with cancer (high, 45.2% mortality; medium, 28.0%; low, 12.1%; $p = 0.008$). Patients with hematologic malignancies had higher median viral loads (CT = 25.0) than patients without cancer (CT = 29.2; $p = 0.0039$). SARS-CoV-2 viral load results may offer vital prognostic information for patients with and without cancer who are hospitalised with COVID-19 [74]. Furthermore, Zitvogel and colleagues analysed data from three prospective cohorts in France and Canada comprising nearly 1,000 individuals. Roughly 50 percent of the participants had cancer. In all three cohorts, the researchers found that patients with cancer had longer SARS-CoV-2 viral shedding compared with cancer-free individuals [75]. Another retrospective study [76] compared 70 patients with SM with 35 HM patients. HM took almost twice as long to reach $C_t > 30$ (HR 1.71, 95% CI [1.004–2.9]) or negativity (HR 2.34 [1.1–5.1]). Interestingly, the maximal viral load in nasopharyngeal swabs, shown to correlate with disease severity and survival [77], was not elevated in patients with HM compared with patients with SM or immunocompetent hosts [78, 79]. Another retrospective study was conducted at Levine Cancer Institute on cancer patients with documented SARS-CoV-2 infection and measurement of viral shedding. Using univariate analysis, the authors found no difference between patients with prolonged shedding versus those shedding less than 30 days for age, gender, race, ethnicity, underlying malignancy, and co-morbidities including body mass index, diabetes, chronic lung conditions, hypertension, or receipt of cytotoxic chemotherapy. They found that presence of symptoms at any point during SARS-CoV-2 infection was associated with prolonged shedding through multivariable analysis. They suggested that symptomatic SARS-CoV-2 infection is associated with prolonged viral shedding in cancer patients when compared with cancer patients with asymptomatic SARS-CoV-2 infection [80]. Another study was carried out on 48 patients diagnosed with solid tumours and COVID-19 from 1 March 2020 to 30 November 2020, at Hospital Universitario Infanta Leonor, Madrid, Spain. Among them, 29 patients received chemotherapy, one patient immunotherapy, and 18 patients other treatments as targeted therapy or radiotherapy. The most predominant histology was lung cancer and breast cancer. Seven patients (14.6%) had localised disease, compared to 41 patients (85.4%) with locally advanced or metastatic disease. Only three patients received convalescent plasma transfusion and 24 specific treatments for COVID-19 (50.0%) (dexamethasone, hydroxychloroquine, lopinavir/ritonavir or remdesivir). Only one patient was admitted to the Intensive Care Unit (ICU) due to the severity of COVID-19. The authors observed that patients with advanced cancer at COVID-19 diagnosis have a greater risk of continuing to present positive RT-PCR with prolonged COVID-19 symptoms, similar to that observed in haematological patients undergoing transplant or CAR T cell therapy [81]. In addition, the authors observed that these patients with advanced disease have the worst prognosis, like lung cancer patients and hematologic cancer patients. The advanced state of immunosuppression induced by their cancer and by the specific oncological treatments received could justify these findings (81). In a further retrospective cohort study, 71 patients were included and 59% of them had a solid tumour, with breast cancer being the most prevalent diagnosis. The median number of days from symptom onset to viral clearance was 37 days with viral load rapidly declining in the first 7–10 days after symptom onset. Within 30 days of diagnosis, 29 (41%) patients were hospitalised and 12 (17%) died. In conclusion, the authors observed that cancer patients, particularly those with multiple comorbidities, had high risk of poor outcomes from COVID-19 with prolonged viral shedding [82].

In summary, patients with cancer, especially those with haematological malignancies or metastatic disease, may be at higher risk for severe COVID-19 because the virus exacerbates their lymphopenia through a variety of different mechanisms that, in turn, can perpetuate viral replication, increase the viral load, and impede the elimination of the virus, which can ultimately result in worse outcomes.

Long-Term COVID-19 Sequelae in Cancer Patients

Many COVID-19 patients after healing can develop the post-COVID-19 syndrome [83], a complex manifestation of likely immune-inflammatory pathogenesis that is characterised by several symptoms, including persistent fatigue, neuro-cognitive sequelae, and varying degrees of respiratory impairment. Recent evidence from the OnCovid study highlighted that more than 1 in 6 cancer patients experiences long-term sequelae following SARS-CoV-2 infection, placing them at increased risk of discontinuing their cancer treatment or dying [84]. Furthermore, this study showed that the 15% of cancer patients who had long-term COVID-19 complications were 76% more likely to die than those without sequelae. Furthermore, these patients were significantly more likely to permanently stop taking their systemic anticancer therapy, and they were more than 3.5 times more likely to die than those who continued their treatment as planned. In terms of long-term complications, almost half of patients experienced dyspnea, and two fifths reported chronic fatigue. Furthermore, the authors noted that COVID-19 sequelae in patients with cancer appear to occur slightly less frequently compared to estimates in the general population – which range from 13% to 60% – though patients with cancer tend to have more respiratory problems. However, it was difficult to compare sequelae rates between cancer patients and the general population because cancer patients could not associate symptoms such as dyspnea and fatigue to long COVID. Furthermore, this study included 1,557 of 2,634 patients who had undergone a clinical reassessment after recovering from COVID-19. The most common cancer diagnoses in this analysis were breast cancer (23.4%), gastrointestinal tumours (16.5%), gynecologic/genitourinary tumours (19.3%), and hematologic cancers (14.1%), with even distribution between local/locoregional and advanced disease. The median interval between COVID-19 recovery and reassessment was 44 days, and the mean post-COVID-19 follow-up period was 128 days. Fifteen percent of patients experienced at least one long-term sequela from COVID-19. The most common were dyspnea/shortness of breath (49.6%), fatigue (41.0%), chronic cough (33.8%), and other respiratory complications (10.7%). Furthermore, the authors noted that cancer patients who experienced sequelae were more likely to be male, aged 65 years or older, to have at least two comorbidities, and to have a history of smoking. In addition, cancer patients who experienced long-term complications were significantly more likely to have had COVID-19 complications, to have required COVID-19 therapy, and to have been hospitalised for the disease. Further analysis of patterns of systemic anticancer therapy in 471 patients revealed that 14.8% of COVID-19 survivors permanently discontinued therapy and that a dose or regimen adjustment occurred for 37.8%. Patients who permanently discontinued anticancer therapy were more likely to be former or current smokers, to have had COVID-19 complications or been hospitalised for COVID-19, and to have had COVID-19 sequelae at reassessment. The investigators found no association between permanent discontinuation of therapy and cancer disease stage. Cortellini and colleagues reported that permanent cessation of systemic anticancer therapy was associated with an increased risk for death. The most common reason for stopping therapy permanently was deterioration of the patient's performance status (61.3%), followed by disease progression (29.0%). Dose or regimen adjustments typically occurred to avoid immune suppression (50.0%), hospitalisation (25.8%), and intravenous drug administration (19.1%). The authors concluded his presentation by highlighting the importance of increasing awareness of long COVID in patients with cancer as well as early treatment of COVID-19 sequelae to improve patient outcomes [84]. In another study, researchers analysed 312 cancer patients and identified 188 cancer patients with long COVID-19 symptoms with a median duration of 7 months and up to 14 months after COVID-19 diagnosis. The most common cancers were skin (seen in 21.9% of the cancer patients), breast (17.7%), prostate (8.3%), lymphoma (8%) and leukemia (5.7%). The most common symptoms reported included fatigue, sleep disturbances, myalgias, and gastrointestinal symptoms, followed by headache, altered smell or taste, dyspnea, and cough [85]. Another study reported that a large proportion (22%) of cancer patients experienced persistent symptoms for more than 6 months after mild disease. In the spectrum of long-lasting signs in cancer cohort, fatigue was the dominant symptom along with neurosensory dysfunction, muscle or joint pain, or respiratory signs, particularly in females and patients with higher body mass index (BMI) [86]. Two studies, using a nationally representative sample of over 4.3 million COVID-19 patients from the National COVID Cohort Collaborative (N3C), described characteristics of patients with cancer and long COVID. The first analysis, among 398,579 adult cancer patients, identified 63,413 (15.9%) COVID-19-positive patients. COVID-19 positivity was significantly correlated with increased risk of all-cause mortality (hazard ratio, 1.20; 95% CI, 1.15 to 1.24). The patients with COVID-19 (age ≥ 65 years, male gender, Southern or Western US residence, an adjusted Charlson Comorbidity Index score ≥ 4) and hematologic malignancy or multitumour sites during cytotoxic therapy had high risk of all-cause mortality [87]. In the second study, a total of 1,700 adult patients with long COVID were identified from the N3C cohort; 634 (37.3%) were cancer patients and 1,066 were non-cancer controls. The most common represented cancers were skin (21.9%), breast (17.7%), prostate (8.3%), lymphoma (8.0%), and leukemia (5.7%). Median age of long-COVID cancer patients was 64 years (Interquartile Range: 54–72), 48.6% were 65 years or older, 60.4% females, 76.8% non-Hispanic White, 12.3% were Black, and 3% Hispanic. A total of 41.1% were current or former smokers, 27.7% had an adjusted Charlson Comorbidity Index score of 0, 18.6% score of 1, and 11.2% score of 2. A total of 57.2% were hospitalised for their initial COVID-19 infection, the average length of stay in the hospital was 9.6 days (SD: 16.7 days), 9.1% required invasive ventilation, and 13% had acute kidney injury during hospitalisation. The most common diagnosis among the non-cancer long COVID patients was asthma (26%), diabetes (17%), chronic kidney disease (12%), heart failure (9.4%), and chronic obstructive pulmonary disease (7.8%). Among long COVID patients, compared to non-cancer controls, cancer patients were more likely to be older (OR = 2.4, 95%CI: 1.1–5.4, p = 0.03), have comorbidities (OR = 4.3, 95%CI: 2.9–6.2, p < 0.0001), and to be hospitalised for COVID-19 (OR = 1.3, 95%CI: 1.0–1.7, p = 0.05), adjusting for sex, race/ethnicity, body mass index, and smoking history. In a nationally representative sample of long COVID patients, there was a relative overrepresentation of patients with cancer. Compared to non-cancer controls, cancer patients were older, more likely to have more comorbidities, and to be hospitalised for COVID-19 [88]. Another study was conducted through telephone survey on 80 cancer patients with confirmed COVID-19 diagnosis [89]. The authors compared patients whose symptoms occurred/got worse more than 4 weeks after COVID-19 diagnosis (classified as long COVID) with patients who did not develop symptoms or whose symptoms occurred/got worse in the first 4 weeks after diagnosis. The authors found that over half of the cancer patients (51.3%; n = 41) developed long COVID with different symptoms such as fatigue, breathlessness, cognitive impairment, sleep disturbance, loss of taste, and depression. In addition, patients who developed long COVID were more likely to undergo neoadjuvant and palliative treatment when compared with those who did not develop long COVID. Moreover, patients who required oxygen therapy and were inpatients at the time of COVID-19 diagnosis were more likely to develop long COVID [89]. The same symptoms were described in a large cohort study by Huang et al [90]. Moreover, a cohort of patients followed for 9 months after COVID-19 infection showed that 30% of patients had persistent symptoms, above all fatigue. Furthermore, patients with severe COVID-19 reported respiratory symptoms (i.e., cough and breathlessness) and loss of taste [91]. This is consistent with the chronic symptoms reported by cancer patients in the current study, where over 80% of patients had severe COVID-19 pneumonia. In addition, the authors found that cancer such as breast, lung, and CNS were associated with long COVID, whereas no significant correlations were found between stage of disease and incidence of long COVID as shown in the study by Pinato et al. [92]. The prolonged effects of COVID infections in cancer patients can be linked to several biological factors of malignant disease. For example, cancer is characterised by impaired autophagy processes [93], which could lead to the accumulation of unfolded proteins in tissues, cellular stress, and inflammation. Several proteins of the COVID-19 virus can interact with the autophagy pathway [94]. Since autophagy is a defective process in cancer, it is possible that an accumulation of viral proteins and other products could potentially prolong viral burden and thus inflammatory processes in tissues of COVID-survivor patients with cancer [95]. However, the data are limited on the effect of post-COVID syndrome in cancer patients since there is an absence of periodic and pre-planned diagnostic tests for sequelae assessment, but these studies provide informative evidence about the long-term effects of COVID-19 in this population.

CREDIT AUTHORSHIP CONTRIBUTION STATEMENT

Gabriella Marfe: Conceptualisation, formal analysis, methodology, visualisation, writing – original draft, – review, and editing. **Stefania Perna and Arvind Kumar Shukla**: Writing – original draft, – review, and editing. **Giovanna Mirone**: Writing – review and editing.

DECLARATION OF COMPETING INTEREST

The authors declare that they have no known competing financial interests or personal relationships that could have appeared to influence the work reported in this chapter.

ACKNOWLEDGMENT

This chapter was not supported by a grant.

REFERENCES

1. Zhou P, Yang X, Wang X, Hu B, Zhang L, Zhang W, et al. A pneumonia outbreak associated with a new coronavirus of probable bat origin. *Nature* 2020;579:270–273. doi: 10.1038/s41586-020-2951-z.
2. World Health Organization: WHO coronavirus (COVID-19) dashboard. (2022). Accessed: May 13, 2022; https://covid19.who.int.
3. Aristodemou K, Buchhass L, Claringbould D. The COVID-19 crisis in the EU: The resilience of healthcare systems, government responses and their socio-economic effects. *Eurasian Econ Rev* 2021;11:251–281 https://doi.org/10.1007/s40822-020-00162.
4. European Commission. (2020d). Communication from the Commission on the implementation of the Green Lanes under the Guidelines for border management measures to protect health and ensure the availability of goods and essential services. COM (2020) 1897 final.
5. Bora VR, Patel BM. The deadly duo of COVID-19 and cancer! *Front Mol Biosci* 2021;8:643004. doi: 10.3389/fmolb.2021.643004.
6. Liang W, Guan W, Chen R, Wang W, Li J, Xu K, et al. Cancer patients in SARS-CoV-2 infection: A nationwide analysis in China. *Lancet Oncol* 2020;21(3):335–337. doi: 10.1016/S1470-2045(20)30096-6.
7. Desai A, Sachdeva S, Parekh T, Desai R. COVID-19 and cancer: Lessons from a pooled meta-analysis. *JCO Glob Oncol.* 2020;6:557–559. doi: 10.1200/GO.20.00097.
8. Zhang L, Zhu F, Xie L, Wang C, Wang J, Chen R, et al. Clinical characteristics of COVID-19-infected cancer patients: A retrospective case study in three hospitals within Wuhan. *China Ann Oncol.* 2020;31(7):894–901. doi: 10.1016/j.annonc.2020.03.296.
9. Mehta V, Goel S, Kabarriti R, Cole D, Goldfinger M, Acuna-Villaorduna A, et al. Case fatality rate of cancer patients with COVID-19 in a New York hospital system. *Cancer Discov.* 2020;10(7):935–941. doi: 10.1158/2159-8290.CD-20-0516.
10. Yu J, Ouyang W, Chua MLK, Xie C. SARS-CoV-2 transmission in patients with cancer at a tertiary care hospital in Wuhan, China. *JAMA Oncol.* 2020;6(7):1108–1110. doi:10.1001/jamaoncol.2020.0980.

11. Bhattacharjee A, Patil VM, Dikshit R, Prabhash K, Singh A, Chaturvedi P. Should we wait or not? The preferable option for patients with stage IV oral cancer in COVID-19 pandemic. *Head Neck.*2020;42(6):1173–1178. doi:0.1002/hed.26196.

12. Wang Y, Grunewald M, Perlman S. Coronaviruses: An updated overview of their replication and pathogenesis. *Methods Mol Biol.* 2020;2203:1–29. doi: 10.1007/978-1-0716-0900-2_1.

13. Sun J, Xiao J, Sun R, Tang X, Liang C, Lin H, et al. Prolonged persistence of SARS-CoV-2 RNA in body fluids. *Emerg Infect Dis.* 2020;26(8):1834–1838. doi: 10.3201/eid2608.201097.

14. Judson SD, Munster VJ. A framework for nosocomial transmission of emerging coronaviruses. *Infect Control Hosp Epidemiol.* 2021 May;42(5):639–641. doi: 10.1017/ice.2020.296.

15. Fu Y, Han P, Zhu R, Bai T, Yi J, Zhao X, et al. Risk factors for viral RNA shedding in COVID-19 patients. *Eur Respir J.* 2020;56(1):2001190. doi: 10.1183/13993003.01190-2020.

16. Qian GQ, Chen XQ, Lv DF, Ma AHY, Wang LP, Yang NB, Duration of SARS-CoV-2 viral shedding during COVID-19 infection. *Infect Dis.* 2020;52(7):511–512. doi: 10.1080/23744235.2020.1748705.

17. Liu Y, Chen X, Zou X, Luo H. A severe-type COVID-19 case with prolonged virus shedding. *J Formos Med Assoc.* 2020;119(10):1555–1557. doi: 10.1016/j.jfma.2020.05.004.

18. Lee S, Kim T, Lee E, Lee C, Kim H, Rhee H, et al. Clinical course and molecular viral shedding among asymptomatic and symptomatic patients with SARS-CoV-2 infection in a community treatment center in the Republic of Korea. *JAMA Intern Med.* 2020;180(11):1447–1452. doi: 10.1001/jamainternmed.2020.3862.

19. Long QX, Tang XJ, Shi QL, Li Q, Deng HJ, Yuan J, et al. Clinical and immunological assessment of asymptomatic SARS-CoV-2 infections. *Nat Med.* 2020;26(8):1200–1204. doi: 10.1038/s41591-020-0965-6.

20. Zou L, Ruan F, Huang M, Liang L, Huang H, Hong Z, et al. SARS-CoV-2 viral load in upper respiratory specimens of infected patients. *N Engl J Med.* 2020;382(12):1177–1179. doi: 10.1056/NEJMc2001737.

21. Li J, Zhang L, Liu B, Song D. Case report: Viral shedding for 60 days in a woman with COVID-19. *Am J Trop Med Hyg.* 2020;102(6):1210–1213. doi: 10.4269/ajtmh.20-0275.

22. Liu WD, Chang SY, Wang JT, Tsai MJ, Hung CC, Hsu CL, et al. Prolonged virus shedding even after seroconversion in a patient with COVID-19. *J Infect.* 2020;81(2):318–356. doi: 10.1016/j.jinf.2020.03.063.

23. Lan L, Xu D, Ye G, Xia C, Wang S, Li Y, Xu H. Positive RT-PCR test results in patients recovered from COVID-19. *JAMA.* 2020;323(15):1502–1503. doi: 10.1001/jama.2020.2783.

24. Hu Z, Song C, Xu C, Jin G, Chen Y, Xu X, et al. Clinical characteristics of 24 asymptomatic infections with COVID-19 screened among close contacts in Nanjing, China. *Sci China. Life Sci.* 2020:706–711. doi: 10.1007/s11427-020-1661-4.

25. He X, Lau EHY, Wu P, Deng X, Wang J, Hao X, et al. Temporal dynamics in viral shedding and transmissibility of COVID-19. *Nat Med.* 2020;26(5):672–675. doi: 10.1038/s41591-020-0869-5.

26. Wölfel R, Corman VM, Guggemos W, Seilmaier M, Zange S, Müller MA, et al. Virological assessment of hospitalized patients with COVID-2019. *Nature.* 2020;581(7809):465–469. doi: 10.1038/s41586-020-2196-x.

27. Bullard J, Dust K, Funk D, Strong JE, Alexander D, Garnett L, et al. Predicting infectious severe acute respiratory syndrome coronavirus 2 from diagnostic samples. *Clin Infect Dis.* 2020;71(10):2663–2666. doi: 10.1093/cid/ciaa638.

28. van Kampen JJA, van de Vijver DAMC, Fraaij PLA, Haagmans BL, Lamers MM, Okba N, et al. Duration and key determinants of infectious virus shedding in hospitalized patients with coronavirus disease-2019 (COVID-19). *Nat Commun.* 2021;12(1):267. doi: 10.1038/s41467-020-20568-4.

29. Dergham J, Delerce J, Bedotto M, La Scola B, Moal V. Isolation of viable SARS-CoV-2 virus from feces of an immunocompromised patient suggesting a possible fecal mode of transmission. *J Clin Med.* 2021;10(12):2696. doi: 10.3390/jcm10122696.

30. Parasa S, Desai M, Thoguluva Chandrasekar V, Patel HK, Kennedy KF, Roesch T, et al. Prevalence of gastrointestinal symptoms and fecal viral shedding in patients with coronavirus disease 2019: A systematic review and meta-analysis. *JAMA Netw Open.* 2020;3(6):e2011335. doi: 10.1001/jamanetworkopen.2020.11335.

31. European Centre for Disease Prevention and Control. Guidance on ending the isolation period for people with COVID-19, third update, 28 January 2022. Stockholm: ECDC; 2022.

32. Cheng HY, Jian SW, Liu DP, Ng TC, Huang WT, Lin HH. Taiwan COVID-19 outbreak investigation team. Contact tracing assessment of COVID-19 transmission dynamics in taiwan and risk at different exposure periods before and after symptom onset. *JAMA Intern Med.* 2020;180(9):1156–1163. doi: 10.1001/jamainternmed.2020.2020.

33. Wei WE, Li Z, Chiew CJ, Yong SE, Toh MP, Lee VJ. Presymptomatic transmission of SARS-CoV-2 – Singapore, January 23–March 16, 2020. *MMWR Morb Mortal Wkly Rep.* 2020;69(14):411–415. doi: 10.15585/mmwr.mm6914e1.

34. Arons MM, Hatfield KM, Reddy SC, Kimball A, James A, Jacobs JR, et al. Public health – Seattle and king county and CDC COVID-19 investigation team. Presymptomatic SARS-CoV-2 infections and transmission in a skilled nursing facility. *N Engl J Med.* 2020;382(22):2081–2090. doi: 10.1056/NEJMoa2008457.

35. Lavezzo E, Franchin E, Ciavarella C, Cuomo-Dannenburg G, Barzon L, Del Vecchio C, Imperial college COVID-19 response team. Suppression of a SARS-CoV-2 outbreak in the Italian municipality of Vo'. *Nature.* 2020;584(7821):425–429. doi: 10.1038/s41586-020-2488-1.

36. Casey-Bryars M, Griffin J, McAloon C, Byrne A, Madden J, Mc Evoy D, et al. Presymptomatic transmission of SARS-CoV-2 infection: A secondary analysis using published data. *BMJ Open.* 2021;11(6):e041240. doi: 10.1136/bmjopen-2020-041240.

37. La Scola B, Le Bideau M, Andreani J, Hoang VT, Grimaldier C, Colson P, et al. Viral RNA load as determined by cell culture as a management tool for discharge of SARS-CoV-2 patients from infectious disease wards. *Eur J Clin Microbiol Infect Dis.* 2020;39(6):1059–1061. doi: 10.1007/s10096-020-03913-9. Epub 2020 April 27. PMID: 32342252.

38. Signorini L, Dolci M, Castelnuovo N, Crespi L, Incorvaia B, Bagnoli P, Parapini S, Basilico N, Galli C, Ambrogi F, Pariani E, Binda S, Ticozzi R, Ferrante P, Delbue S. Longitudinal, virological, and serological assessment of hospitalized COVID-19 patients. *J Neurovirol.* 2022 Feb;28(1):113–122. doi: 10.1007/s13365-021-01029-0.

39. ASCO special report: Guide to cancer care delivery during the COVID-19 pandemic. Available at: https://www.asco.org/sites/new-www.asco.org/files/content-files/2020-ASCO-Guide-Cancer-COVID19.pdf. Accessed September 9, 2020.

40. Lee LY, Cazier JB, Angelis V, Arnold R, Bisht V, Campton NA, et al. UK coronavirus monitoring project team, Kerr R, Middleton G. COVID-19 mortality in patients with

cancer on chemotherapy or other anticancer treatments: A prospective cohort study. *Lancet.* 2020;395(10241):1919–1926. doi: 10.1016/S0140-6736(20)31173-9.

41. Wong W, Brieva C, May M, Gambina K, Whittier S, Hod EA, et al. A double-edged sword: Prolonged detection of SARS-COV-2 in patients receiving cancer directed therapy. *Semin Oncol.* 2021;48(2):166–170. doi: 10.1053/j.seminoncol.2020.11.001.

42. Bakouny Z, Hawley JE, Choueiri TK, Peters S, Rini BI, Warner JL, et al. COVID-19 and cancer: Current challenges and perspectives. *Cancer Cell.* 2020;38(5):629–646. doi: 10.1016/j.ccell.2020.09.018.

43. García LF. Immune response, inflammation, and the clinical spectrum of COVID-19. *Front Immunol.* 2020; 11:1441. doi: 10.3389/fimmu.2020.01441.

44. Zhou F, Yu T, Du R, Fan G, Liu Y, Liu Z, et al. Clinical course and risk factors for mortality of adult inpatients with COVID-19 in Wuhan, China: A retrospective cohort study. *Lancet.* 2020;395(10229):1054–1062. https://doi.org/10.1016/S0140-6736(20)30566-3.

45. Elkrief A, Wu JT, Jani C, Enriquez KT, Glover M, Shah MR, et al. Learning through a pandemic: The current state of knowledge on COVID-19 and cancer. *Cancer Discov.* 2022;12(2):303–330. doi: 10.1158/2159-8290.CD-21-1368.

46. Tembhare PR, Sriram H, Chatterjee G, Khanka T, Gokarn A, Mirgh S, et al. Comprehensive immune cell profiling depicts an early immune response associated with severe coronavirus disease 2019 in cancer patients. *Immunol Cell Biol.* 2022;100(1):61–73. doi: 10.1111/imcb.12504.

47. Kwon G, Kim HJ, Park SJ, Lee HE, Woo H, et al. Anxiolytic-like effect of danshensu [(3-(3,4-dihydroxyphenyl)-lactic acid)] in mice. *Life Sci.* 2014;101(1–2):73–78. doi: 10.1016/j.lfs.2014.02.011.

48. Esperança-Martins M, Gonçalves L, Soares-Pinho I, Gomes A, Serrano M, Blankenhaus B, et al. Humoral immune response of SARS-CoV-2-infected patients with cancer: Influencing factors and mechanisms. *Oncologist.* 2021;26(9):e1619 –e1632. doi: 10.1002/onco.13828.

49. Hu B, Huang S, Yin L. The cytokine storm and COVID-19. *J Med Virol.* 2021;93(1):250–256. doi: 10.1002/jmv.26232.

50. RECOVERY Collaborative Group, Horby P, Lim WS, Emberson JR, Mafham M, Bell JL, Linsell L, et al. Dexamethasone in hospitalized patients with Covid-19. *N Engl J Med.* 2021;384(8):693–704. doi: 10.1056/NEJMoa2021436.

51. Fendler A, Au L, Shepherd STC, Byrne F, Cerrone M, Boos LA, et al. CAPTURE consortium. Functional antibody and T cell immunity following SARS-CoV-2 infection, including by variants of concern, in patients with cancer: The CAPTURE study. *Nat Cancer.* 2021;2(12):1321–1337. doi: 10.1038/s43018-021-00275-9.

52. Bange EM, Han NA, Wileyto P, Kim JY, Gouma S, Robinson J, et al. CD8+T cells contribute to survival in patients with COVID-19 and hematologic cancer. *Nat Med.* 2021;27(7):1280–1289. doi: 10.1038/s41591-021-01386-7.

53. Abdul-Jawad S, Baù L, Alaguthurai T, Del Molino Del Barrio I, Laing AG, et al. Acute immune signatures and their legacies in severe acute respiratory syndrome coronavirus-2 infected cancer patients. *Cancer Cell.* 2021;39(2):257–275.e6. doi: 10.1016/j.ccell.2021.01.001.

54. Nakajima Y, Ogai A, Furukawa K, Arai R, Anan R, Nakano Y, et al. Prolonged viral shedding of SARS-CoV-2 in an immunocompromised patient. *J Infect Chemother.* 2021 Februry;27(2):387–389. doi: 10.1016/j.jiac.2020.12.001.

55. Hoffmann M, Kleine-Weber H, Schroeder S, Krüger N, Herrler T, Erichsen S, et al. SARS-CoV-2 cell entry depends on ACE2 and TMPRSS2 and is blocked by a clinically proven protease inhibitor. *Cell.* 2020;181(2):271–280. doi: 10.1016/j.cell.2020.02.052.

56. Krämer B, Knoll R, Bonaguro L, ToVinh M, Raabe J, Astaburuaga-García R, Schulte-Schrepping J, Kaiser KM, Rieke GJ, Bischoff J, Monin MB, Hoffmeister C, Schlabe S, De Domenico E, Reusch N, Händler K, Reynolds G, Blüthgen N, Hack G, Finnemann C, Nischalke HD, Strassburg CP, Stephenson E, Su Y, Gardner L, Yuan D, Chen D, Goldman J, Rosenstiel P, Schmidt SV, Latz E, Hrusovsky K, Ball AJ, Johnson JM, Koenig PA, Schmidt FI, Haniffa M, Heath JR, Kümmerer BM, Keitel V, Jensen B, Stubbemann P, Kurth F, Sander LE, Sawitzki B; Deutsche COVID-19 OMICS Initiative (DeCOI); Aschenbrenner AC, Schultze JL, Nattermann J. Early IFN-α signatures and persistent dysfunction are distinguishing features of NK cells in severe COVID-19. *Immunity.* 2021; Nov 9;54(11):2650–2669. doi: 10.1016/j.immuni.2021.09.002.

57. Goubet AG, Dubuisson A, Geraud A, Danlos FX, Terrisse S, Silva CAC, et al. Prolonged SARS-CoV-2 RNA virus shedding and lymphopenia are hallmarks of COVID-19 in cancer patients with poor prognosis. *Cell Death Differ.* 2021;28(12):3297–3315. doi: 10.1038/s41418-021-00817-9.

58. Aydillo T, Gonzalez-Reiche AS, Aslam S, van de Guchte A, Khan Z, Obla A, et al. Shedding of viable SARS-CoV-2 after immunosuppressive therapy for cancer. *N Engl J Med.* 2020;383(26):2586–2588. doi: 10.1056/NEJMc203167.

59. Roel E, Pistillo A, Recalde M, Fernández-Bertolín S, Aragón M, Soerjomataram I, Jenab M, et al. Cancer and the risk of coronavirus disease 2019 diagnosis, hospitalisation and death: A population-based multistate cohort study including 4 618 377 adults in Catalonia, *Spain. Int J Cancer* 2022;150(5):782–794. doi: 10.1002/ijc.33846.

60. Fontana LM, Villamagna AH, Sikka MK, McGregor JC. Understanding viral shedding of severe acute respiratory coronavirus virus 2 (SARS-CoV-2): Review of current literature. *Infect Control Hosp Epidemiol.* 2021;42(6):659–668. doi: 10.1017/ice.2020.1273.

61. Walker AS, Pritchard E, House T, Robotham JV, Birrell PJ, Bell I, et al. COVID-19 Infection survey team. C_t threshold values, a proxy for viral load in community SARS-CoV-2 cases, demonstrate wide variation across populations and over time. *Elife.* 2021;10:e64683. doi: 10.7554/eLife.64683.

62. Arcani R, Colle J, Cauchois R, Koubi M, Jarrot PA, Jean R, et al. Clinical characteristics and outcomes of patients with haematologic malignancies and COVID-19 suggest that prolonged SARS-CoV-2 carriage is an important issue. *Ann Hematol.* 2021;100(11):2799–2803. doi: 10.1007/s00277-021-04656-z. Epub 2021 September 13.

63. Belsky JA, Tullius BP, Lamb MG, Sayegh R, Stanek JR, Auletta JJ. COVID-19 in immunocompromised patients: A systematic review of cancer, hematopoietic cell and solid organ transplant patients. *J Infect.* 2021;82(3):329–338. doi: 10.1016/j.jinf.2021.01.022.

64. Duléry R, Lamure S, Delord M, Di Blasi R, Chauchet A, Hueso T, et al. Prolonged in-hospital stay and higher mortality after COVID-19 among patients with non-Hodgkin lymphoma treated with B-cell depleting immunotherapy. *Am J Hematol.* 2021;96(8):934–944. doi: 10.1002/ajh.26209.

65. Xu K, Chen Y, Yuan J, Yi P, Ding C, Wu W, et al. Factors associated with prolonged viral RNA shedding in patients with coronavirus disease 2019 (COVID-19). *Clin Infect Dis.* 2020 July 28;71(15):799–806. doi: 10.1093/cid/ciaa351.

66. Avanzato VA, Matson MJ, Seifert SN, Pryce R, Williamson BN, Anzick SL, et al. Case study: Prolonged infectious SARS-CoV-2 shedding from an asymptomatic immunocompromised individual with cancer. *Cell.* 2020;183(7):1901–1912. doi: 10.1016/j.cell.2020.10.049.

67. Kaya BS, Yılmam İ, Çakır Edis E, Karabulut D, Elmaslar Mert T, et al. Case of prolonged viral shedding: Chronic, intermittant COVID-19? *Turk Thorac J.* 2022;23(1):85–88. doi: 10.5152/TurkThoracJ.2022.21141.

68. Altamirano-Molina M, Pacheco-Modesto I, Amado-Tineo J. Prolonged viral shedding of SARS-CoV-2 in patients with acute leukemia. *Hematol Transfus Cell Ther.* 2022;44(2):299–300. doi: 10.1016/j.htct.2021.11.017.

69. Lee CY, Shah MK, Hoyos D, Solovyov A, Douglas M, Taur Y, et al. Prolonged SARS-CoV-2 infection in patients with lymphoid malignancies. *Cancer Discov.* 2022;12(1):62–73. doi: 10.1158/2159-8290.CD-21-1033.

70. Martínez-Barranco P, García-Roa M, Trelles-Martínez R, Arribalzaga K, Velasco M, Guijarro C, et al. Management of persistent SARS-CoV-2 infection in patients with follicular lymphoma. *Acta Haematol.* 2022;145(4):384–393. doi: 10.1159/000521121.

71. Berktas BM, Koyuncu A. Case report: Unremitting COVID-19 pneumonia, viral shedding, and failure to develop anti-SARS-CoV-2 antibodies for more than 6 months in patient with mantle cell lymphoma treated with rituximab. *Am J Trop Med Hyg.* 2022;106(4):1104–1107. doi: 10.4269/ajtmh.21-1010.

72. Infante MS, González-Gascón Y, Marín I, Muñoz-Novas C, Churruca J, Foncillas MÁ, et al. COVID-19 in patients with hematological malignancies: A retrospective case series. *Int J Lab Hematol.* 2020;42(6):e256–e259. doi: 10.1111/ijlh.13301.

73. Nagai H, Saito M, Adachi E, Sakai-Tagawa Y, Yamayoshi S, Kiso M, Kawamata T, et al. Casirivimab/imdevimab for active COVID-19 pneumonia which persisted for nine months in a patient with follicular lymphoma during anti-CD20 therapy. *Jpn J Infect Dis.* 2022 November 22;75(6):608–611. doi: 10.7883/yoken.JJID.2022.092.

74. Westblade LF, Brar G, Pinheiro LC, Paidoussis D, Rajan M, Martin P, et al. SARS-CoV-2 viral load predicts mortality in patients with and without cancer who are hospitalized with COVID-19. *Cancer Cell.* 2020;38(5):661–671.e2. doi: 10.1016/j.ccell.2020.09.007.

75. Goubet AG, Dubuisson A, Geraud A, Danlos FX, Terrisse S, Silva CAC, Drubay D, Touri L, Picard M, Mazzenga M, Silvin A, Dunsmore G, Haddad Y, Pizzato E, Ly P, Flament C, Melenotte C, Solary E, Fontenay M, Garcia G, Balleyguier C, Lassau N, Maeurer M, Grajeda-Iglesias C, Nirmalathasan N, Aprahamian F, Durand S, Kepp O, Ferrere G, Thelemaque C, Lahmar I, Fahrner JE, Meziani L, Ahmed-Belkacem A, Saïdani N, La Scola B, Raoult D, Gentile S, Cortaredona S, Ippolito G, Lelouvier B, Roulet A, Andre F, Barlesi F, Soria JC, Pradon C, Gallois E, Pommeret F, Colomba E, Ginhoux F, Kazandjian S, Elkrief A, Routy B, Miyara M, Gorochov G, Deutsch E, Albiges L, Stoclin A, Gachot B, Florin A, Merad M, Scotte F, Assaad S, Kroemer G, Blay JY, Marabelle A, Griscelli F, Zitvogel L, Derosa L. Prolonged SARS-CoV-2 RNA virus shedding and lymphopenia are hallmarks of COVID-19 in cancer patients with poor prognosis. *Cell Death Differ.* 2021;28(12):3297–3315. doi: 10.1038/s41418-021-00817-9.

76. Babady NE, Cohen B, McClure T, Chow K, Caldararo M, Jani K, et al. Variable duration of viral shedding in cancer patients with coronavirus disease 2019 (COVID-19). *Infect Control Hosp Epidemiol.* 2021:1–3. doi: 10.1017/ice.2021.378.

77. Kawasuji H, Morinaga Y, Tani H, Yoshida Y, Takegoshi Y, Kaneda M, et al. SARS-CoV-2 RNAemia with a higher nasopharyngeal viral load is strongly associated with disease severity and mortality in patients with COVID-19. *J Med Virol.* 2022;94(1):147–153. doi: 10.1002/jmv.27282.

78. Barbui T, De Stefano V, Alvarez-Larran A, Iurlo A, Masciulli A, Carobbio A, et al. Among classic myeloproliferative neoplasms, essential thrombocythemia is

associated with the greatest risk of venous thromboembolism during COVID-19. *Blood Cancer J.* 2021;11(2):21. doi: 10.1038/s41408-021-00417-3.

79. Fox-Lewis A, Fox-Lewis S, Beaumont J, Drinković D, Harrower J, Howe K,et al. SARS-CoV-2 viral load dynamics and real-time RT-PCR cycle threshold interpretation in symptomatic non-hospitalised individuals in New Zealand: A multicentre cross sectional observational study. *Pathology.* 2021;53(4):530–535. doi: 10.1016/j.pathol.2021.01.007.

80. Shahid Z, Baldrige E, Trufan S, Schepel C, Tan AR, Hwang JJ, et al. Upper respiratory tract SARS-CoV-2 viral shedding in cancer patients *J Clin Onco* 2021;39(15):e18776–e18776.

81. Rogado J, Gullón P, Obispo B, Serrano G, Lara MÁ. Prolonged SARS-CoV-2 viral shedding in patients with solid tumours and associated factors. *Eur J Cancer.* 2021;148:58–60. doi: 10.1016/j.ejca.2021.02.011.

82. Yoke LH, Lee JM, Krantz EM, Morris J, Marquis S, Bhattacharyya P, et al. Clinical and virologic characteristics and outcomes of coronavirus disease 2019 at a cancer center. *Open Forum Infect Dis.* 2021 April 16;8(6):ofab193. doi: 10.1093/ofid/ofab193.

83. Sandler CX, Wyller VBB, Moss-Morris R, Buchwald D, Crawley E, Hautvast J, et al. Long COVID and post-infective fatigue syndrome: A review. *Open Forum Infect Dis.* 2021;8(10):ofab440. doi: 10.1093/ofid/ofab440.

84. Cortellini A, Salazar R, Gennari A, Aguilar-Company J, Bower M, Bertuzzi A, et al.; On Covid study group. Persistence of long-term COVID-19 sequelae in patients with cancer: An analysis from the OnCovid registry. *Eur J Cancer.* 2022;170:10–16. doi: 10.1016/j.ejca.2022.03.019.

85. Dagher H, Malek A, Chaftari AN, Subbiahm IM, Jiangm Y, Lamie P, Granwehr B, et al. Long COVID in cancer patients: Preponderance of symptoms in majority of patients over long time period. *Open Forum Infectious Diseases* 2021 November;8(Suppl. 1), S256–S257. doi: https://doi.org/10.1093/ofid/ofab466.502.

86. Hajjaji N, Lepoutre K, Lakhdar S, Bécourt S, Bellier C, Kaczmarek E, et al. 16 months follow up of patients' behavior and mild COVID-19 patterns in a large cohort of cancer patients during the pandemic. *Front Oncol.* 2022;12:901426. doi: 10.3389/fonc.2022.901426.

87. Sharafeldin N, Bates B, Song Q, Madhira V, Yan Y, Dong S, Lee E, Kuhrt N, et al.Outcomes of COVID-19 in patients with cancer: Report from the national COVID cohort collaborative (N3C). *J Clin Oncol.* 2021 July 10;39(20):2232–2246. doi: 10.1200/JCO.21.01074.

88. Sharafeldin N, Madhira V, Song Q, Bates B, Mitra AK, Liu F, et al. Long COVID-19 in patients with cancer: Report from the national COVID cohort collaborative (N3C). *Journal of Clinical Oncology* 2022;40(suppl. 16):1540–1540.

89. Monroy-Iglesias MJ, Tremble K, Russell B, Moss C, Dolly S, Sita-Lumsden A, et al. Long-term effects of COVID-19 on cancer patients: The experience from Guy's Cancer Centre. *Future Oncol.* 2022 October;18(32):3585–3594. doi: 10.2217/fon-2022-0088. Epub 2022 September 29.

90. Huang C, Huang L, Wang Y, Li X, Ren L, Gu X, et al. 6-month consequences of COVID-19 in patients discharged from hospital: A cohort study. *Lancet.* 2021 Jan 16;397(10270):220–232. doi: 10.1016/S0140-6736(20)32656-8.

91. Logue JK, Franko NM, McCulloch DJ, McDonald D, Magedson A, Wolf CR, Chu HY. Sequelae in adults at 6 months after COVID-19 infection. *JAMA Netw Open.* 2021;4(2):e210830. doi: 10.1001/jamanetworkopen.2021.0830. Erratum in: *JAMA Netw Open.* 2021 March 1;4(3):e214572.

92. Pinato DJ, Lee AJX, Biello F, Seguí E, Aguilar-Company J, Carbó A, Bruna R, et al. Presenting features and early mortality from SARS-CoV-2 infection in cancer patients during the initial stage of the COVID-19 pandemic in Europe. *Cancers* 2020 July 8;12(7):1841. doi: 10.3390/cancers12071841.

93. White E. The role for autophagy in cancer. *J Clin Invest.* 2015 January;125(1):42–46. doi: 10.1172/JCI73941. Epub 2015 January 2. PMID: 25654549.

94. Zang R, Gomez Castro MF, McCune BT, Zeng Q, Rothlauf PW, Sonnek NM, et al. TMPRSS2 and TMPRSS4 promote SARS-CoV-2 infection of human small intestinal enterocytes. *Sci Immunol.* 2020 13;5(47):eabc3582. doi: 10.1126/sciimmunol.abc3582.

95. Gaebler C, Wang Z, Lorenzi JCC, Muecksch F, Finkin S, Tokuyama M, et al. Evolution of antibody immunity to SARS-CoV-2. *Nature.* 2021;591(7851):639–644. doi: 10.1038/s41586-021-03207-w.

10

COVID-19 Vaccine Development and Cancer

Kenneth Lundstrom

Introduction

The current COVID-19 pandemic caused by the SARS-CoV-2 has resulted in more than 765 million infections and more than 6.9 million deaths worldwide. Coronaviruses are single-stranded RNA (ssRNA) viruses encapsulated by an envelope structure consisting of various proteins. For instance, SARS-CoV-2 possesses the following structural proteins: nucleocapsid (N), membrane (M), envelope (E), and spike (S) proteins [1]. Especially the S protein has been a prominent target for vaccine development as its function is to bind to the host cell angiotensin-converting enzyme 2 (ACE2) receptor [2]. Therefore, a large number of SARS-CoV-2 vaccine candidates are based on the full-length S protein or some regions thereof such as the receptor binding domain (RBD), as described below. Additionally, based on bioinformatics and structural modelling the SARS-CoV-2 E protein shares sequence similarity with its counterpart in SARS-CoV with a highly conserved N-terminus and the potential of functioning as a gated ion channel conducting H^+ ions [3]. The hydrophobic and central core structures in the E protein may regulate the opening and closing of the channel thereby playing a critical role in viral infection and pathogenesis. Moreover, the five non-structural proteins nsp3 and 3CL-pro, and nsp8, nsp9, and nsp10 of coronaviruses have been predicted to be adhesins, crucial for viral adhesion and host invasion [4].

Due to the urgent need for the development of an efficient vaccine against SARS-CoV-2, more or less all available strategies have been applied as indicated by more than 160 COVID-19 vaccine candidates subjected to preclinical studies and more than 50 vaccine candidates for whom clinical trials have either been conducted or which are currently in progress (www.who.int/publications/m/item/draft-landscape-of-covid-19-candidate-vaccines).

Vaccine Development Strategies for Preclinical Evaluation

Inactivated and live-attenuated vaccines present straightforward approaches for immunisation strategies. Inactivated SARS-CoV-2 has been used as a vaccine candidate generating high levels of neutralising antibodies in mice, rats, guinea pigs, and nonhuman primates [5]. Two immunisations with 2 µg of inactivated

DOI: 10.1201/9781003362562-11

SARS-CoV-2 protected rhesus macaques against intratracheal challenges with SARS-CoV-2. In a study in mice, rats, and macaques, the inactivated SARS-CoV-2 vaccine candidate PiCoVacc induced SARS-CoV-2-specific neutralising antibodies [6].

Protein subunit vaccines have been engineered as capsid-like particles (CLPs) to display the SARS-CoV-2 S RBD, which elicited high levels of neutralising antibodies in mice after only one single immunisation [7]. The titers were comparable with those observed in recovering COVID-19 patients and superior after booster immunisations. In another study, four versions of the S protein, the RBD, the S1 subunit, the wildtype S ectodomain (S-WT), and the prefusion trimer-stabilised form (S-2P) were expressed in Sf9 insect cells [8]. Although the RBD version appeared as a monomer, whereas the three other versions assembled as homotrimers, they all elicited excellent antigenicity. All versions except for S1 induced high neutralisation titres in mice after three injections. Furthermore, S-2P elicited neutralising antibodies in non-human primates, which were more than 40 times higher than those measured in convalescent COVID-19 patients. In another approach, liposomal encapsulation of monomeric or trimeric SARS-CoV-2 S protein and STING agonist adjuvant induced systemic neutralising antibodies, mucosa/l IgA responses in the lung and nasal compartments, and T-cell responses in the lung after a single-dose intranasal administration in mice [9].

Peptide vaccine-based strategies have also been considered for SARS-CoV-2 by an immunoinformatics approach [10]. Thirteen MHC-1 class and three MHC-II class epitopes within the SARS-CoV-2 S protein were identified and could constitute ideal candidates for a multi-epitope peptide vaccine. Furthermore, docking of vaccine candidates with the toll-like receptor 5 (TLR-5) could further support vaccine development and should be evaluated in vitro and in vivo. In another study, B- and T-cell epitopes for SARS-CoV-2 S, M, and N proteins were identified using immunoinformatics approaches [11]. A total of five B-cell epitopes in the RBD of the S protein and seven MHC-I class and 18 MHC-II class binding T-cell epitopes from S, M, and N proteins were identified and will be subjected to vaccine development. In another bioinformatics approach, computational evaluation suggested that a SARS-CoV-2 vaccine candidate consisting of 33 highly antigenic epitopes of the S, M, and N proteins is non-toxic, non-allergenic, thermostable, and elicits humoral and cell-mediated immune responses and potentially may have a prominent role in host-receptor recognition, viral entry, and pathogenicity [12]. Furthermore, based on docking and molecular dynamics, a novel 18 amino acid long peptide was designed to inhibit the interaction of SARS-CoV-2 S with ACE2, resulting in the blocking cellular entry of SARS-CoV-2 [13].

Viral vectors represent a large part of COVID-19 vaccine development both at the preclinical and clinical levels [14]. The viral expression systems employed include for example adenoviruses (Ad), measles viruses (MV), poxviruses, lentiviruses, and rhabdoviruses [14]. Several preclinical studies have demonstrated strong SARS-CoV-2–specific immune responses and protection against challenges with SARS-CoV-2 in animals immunised with viral vector-based vaccine candidates [15–20].

DNA-based vaccines have become attractive due to the easy plasmid DNA handling, manufacturing, and product stability facilitating storage and transport [21].

Several alternative delivery methods for DNA vaccines have been applied, including the administration of naked plasmid DNA [22], electroporation [23], gene gun [24], liposome-based [25], and polymer-based nanoparticles [26]. Plasmid DNA–based safety, expression, and immunogenicity have been improved by the deletion of non-essential bacterial sequences [27], engineering of minicircle DNA [28], the combination of promoters/enhancers and post-translational regulatory elements [29, 30], and codon optimisation [31]. The DNA vaccine INO-4800 expressing the SARS-CoV-2 S protein elicited neutralising antibodies in mice and guinea pigs [32]. Similarly, another DNA–based SARS-CoV-2 S vaccine protected primates against SARS-CoV-2 challenges [33].

RNA-based vaccines present an attractive alternative as the RNA delivered to the cytoplasm will be directly translated in the host cell cytoplasm, resulting in high levels of antigen expression and potentially strong immune responses. On the other hand, single-stranded mRNA is highly sensitive to degradation, which has resulted in efforts to stabilise mRNA by incorporation of anti-reverse cap analogues (ARCAs) [34], engineering of the 5′ and 3′ ends of the mRNA including the poly(A) tail [35], and chemical modifications by the introduction of pseudouridines in the RNA sequence [36]. Another approach has been liposome encapsulation of RNA to improve the delivery and stability of mRNA molecules [37]. An attractive approach has been to utilise RNA replicons of self-amplifying RNA (saRNA) viruses, which can provide a 20,000-fold amplification of RNA in the cytoplasm of transfected cells [38]. For instance, formulations with ionizable C12-200 and cationic DDA and DOTAP lipids produced lipid nanoparticles (LNPs) with both exterior and interior saRNA for efficient delivery [39].

In the context of COVID-19 vaccine development, engineering of prefusion-stabilising mutations of the SARS-COV-2 S trimers, which when delivered as LNP–encapsulated mRNA-1273 elicited potent neutralising antibodies and CD8+ T-cell responses in immunised mice [40]. Moreover, immunisation with LNP-mRNA-1273 protected mice after challenges with SARS-CoV-2 showing no immunopathology in lungs and noses. The mRNA-1273 vaccine candidate has also been evaluated in non-human primates [41]. Immunisation with 10 or 100 µg of mRNA-1273 induced higher antibody levels than observed in sera from convalescent COVID-19 patients. Furthermore, immunisations induced type 1 helper T-cell (Th1)-biased CD4 T-cell responses and low or undetectable Th2 or CD8 T-cell responses. The immunisation also protected primates from pathological changes in the upper and lower airways and in the lungs. Moreover, the BNT162b1 and BNT162b2 vaccine candidates based on LNP–encapsulated SARS-CoV-2 S RBD or full-length mRNA, respectively, have demonstrated protection against challenges with SARS-CoV-2 in immunised macaques [42]. Optimisation of mRNA translation has been achieved by customised 5′ and 3′ end regions, which have been tested for several SARS-CoV-2 constructs [43]. LNP formulations of the lead candidate demonstrated high levels of neutralising antibodies in animal models. Furthermore, the Lipid-enabled and Unlocked Nucleomonomer Agent modified RNA (LUNAR®) multi-component delivery system has provided positive results in preclinical studies for mRNA-based COVID-19 vaccines [44]. In another mRNA-based vaccine approach the mRNA for the SARS-CoV-2 S RBD was encapsulated in LNPs resulting in the ARCoV vaccine candidate [45] (Table 10.1).

TABLE 10.1

Examples of Preclinical SARS-CoV-2 Vaccine Studies

Approach/Vaccine	Target	Response	Ref
Inactivated virus			
BBIBP-CorV	Inactivated SARS-CoV-2	Protection in rhesus macaques	[5, 6]
	Inactivated SARS-CoV-2	Good safety, neutralising antibodies in Phase I	[46]
	Inactivated SARS-CoV-2	Good safety, neutralising antibodies in Phase II	[47]
SinoVac	Inactivated SARS-CoV-2	Good safety, neutralising antibodies in Phase I/II	[48]
	Inactivated SARS-CoV-2	Good safety, vaccine efficacy 83.5%	[49]
	Inactivated SARS-CoV-2	Approval in China	
PiCoVacc	Inactivated SARS-CoV-2	Protection in rhesus macaques	[7]
Protein subunit			
RBD	CLP-SARS-CoV-2 RBD	Strong immune response in mice	[8]
S-WT	MC-SARS-CoV-2	Protection of immunized hamsters	[8]
S-2P	SARS-CoV-2 S regions	40x higher titers than in patients	[8]
S1	SARS-CoV-2 S	Systemic neutralizing antibodies	[8]
NanoSTING-Trimer	SARS-CoV-2 S STING	Intranasal delivery, neutralising antibodies in mice	[9]
NVX-CoV2373	SARS-CoV-2 S	Neutralising antibodies in Phase I	[50]
	SARS-CoV-2 S	Vaccine efficacy 87.5-89.9% in Phase III	[51]
	SARS-CoV-2 S	EUA in the EU and the UK	[53]
ZF2001	SARS.CoV-2 S RBD	Good safety, 97% seroconversion in Phase II	[54]
Peptides			
	SARS-CoV-2 S	Immunoinformatics-based epitope identification	[10]
	SARS-CoV-2 S, M, N	Immunoinformatics on epitopes	[11]
	SARS-CoV-2 S, M, N	Bioinformatics on 33 epitopes	[12]
	SARS-CoV-2 S	18 amino acid-peptide targeting S	[13]
Viral vectors			
AdChOx1	SARS-CoV-2 S	Strong immune response in mice	[15]
	SARS-CoV-2 S	Pneumonia protection in macaques	[16]
	SARS-CoV-2 S	Immune response in Phase I	[66]
	SARS-CoV-2 S	Vaccine efficacy 62.1% in Phase III	[68]
	SARS-CoV-2 S	EUA in the UK	[69]
Ad5	SARS-CoV-2 S	Protection in rhesus macaques	[17]
	SARS-CoV-2 S	Good safety, humoral immune responses in Phase I	[55]
	SARS-CoV-2 S	Good safety, vaccine efficacy 57.5% in Phase III	[58]
	SARS-CoV-2 S	EUA in several countries	[59]
Ad26	SARS-CoV-2 S	Protection in hamsters	[18]
	SARS-CoV-2 S	Protection in rhesus macaques	[19]
	SARS-CoV-2 S	Vaccine efficacy after single injection in Phase I/II	[61]
	SARS-CoV-2 S	Vaccine efficacy 66.9-85.4% in Phase III	[63]
	SARS-CoV-2 S	EUA in the US	
Ad26 + Ad5	rAd26-S/rAd5-S	Vaccine efficacy in animal models	[20]
	rAd26-S/rAd5-S	Vaccine efficacy in Phase III	[65]
	rAd26-S/rAd5-S	Approval in Russia	[64]

(Continued)

TABLE 10.1 (Continued)

Approach/Vaccine	Target	Response	Ref
DNA			
INO-4800	SARS-CoV-2 S	Neutralising antibodies in mice and guinea pigs	[32]
	SARS-CoV-2 S	Good safety, immune responses in Phase I	[70]
	SARS-CoV-2 S	Immune responses in Phase I/II	[71]
DNA-COVID-19	SARS-CoV-2 S	Protection in rhesus macaques	[33]
ZyCoV-D	SARS-CoV-2 S	Good safety, strong immune responses in Phase I	[72]
	SARS-CoV-2 S	Vaccine efficacy of 66.6% in Phase III	[73]
	SARS-CoV-2 S	Approved in India	[74]
RNA			
LNP-RNA1273	SARS-CoV-2 S	Protection in mice	[40]
	SARS-CoV-2 S	Protection in non-human primates	[41]
	SARS-CoV-2 S	Good safety, and immune responses in Phase I	[84]
	SARS-CoV-2 S	Vaccine efficacy of 94.1% in Phase III	[86]
	SARS-CoV-2 S	EUA in the US, Europe	[87]
LNP-BNT162b1/b2	SARS-CoV-2 S/RBD	Protection in macaques	[42]
LNP-BNT162b2	SARS-CoV-2 S	Neutralising antibodies in animal models	[43]
	SARS-CoV-2 S	Good safety, and immunogenicity in Phase I/II	[80]
	SARS-CoV-2 S	Vaccine efficacy of 95% in Phase III	[82]
	SARS-CoV-2 S	EUA in Europe, the UK, and the US	[83]
LUNAR®LNP-mRNA	SARS-CoV-2 S	Positive results in preclinical	[44]
	SARS-CoV-2 S	Good safety and tolerability in Phase I	[76]
ARCoV	SARS-CoV-2 S RBD	Protection in mice, storage at RT	[45]
	SARS-CoV-2 S RBD	Good safety, humoral immune responses in Phase I	[78]
CVnCoV	SARS-CoV-2 S	Good safety, immune responses in Phase I	[79]
LNP-nCoVsaRNA	SARS-CoV-2 S	Good safety, modest immune responses in Phase I	[88]

EUA, Emergency Use Authorization; LNP, lipid nanoparticles; LUNAR®, Lipid-enabled and Unlocked Nucleomonomer Agent modified RNA; M, membrane protein; MC, molecular clamp: N, nucleocapsid protein; RBD, receptor binding domain; S, spike protein; SARS-CoV. Severe Acute Respiratory Syndrome-Coronavirus.

Clinical Trials

Clinical trials on COVID-19 vaccine candidates involve vaccine candidates based on inactivated virus, protein subunits, non-replicating and replicating viral vectors, and nucleic acids, as summarised below.

An **inactivated virus vaccine** candidate has been produced in Vero cells, which has been subjected to a Phase I/II clinical trial [46] (ChiCTR2000031809). The interim report indicated that 96 participants took part in the phase I trial, applying three doses of 2.5, 5, and 10 μg. The phase II trial included 224 adults scheduled for two doses of 5 μg. The study revealed only low-rate adverse reactions and demonstrated neutralising antibody responses in both trial phases. In another randomised, double-blind, placebo-controlled phase I/II trial, 192 and 336 participants were subjected to phase I and phase II trials, respectively, receiving the inactivated SARS-CoV-2 vaccine BBIBP-CorV [47] (ChiCTR2000032459). The phase I study comprised a two-dose schedule of 2, 4, and 8 µg, and individuals in the phase II trial received either a single dose of 8 µg or two administrations of 4 µg. Although some adverse reactions occurred, they were generally mild or moderate. Vaccine-elicited neutralising antibodies were obtained for all doses and humoral responses against SARS-CoV-2 were detected in all vaccinees. Moreover, interim results from a phase I/II trial in 18–59 year-old volunteers with an inactivated SARS-CoV-2 vaccine candidate produced by Sinovac showed good safety and seroconversion of neutralising antibodies [48]. Likewise, among 600 participants in phase II, no severe adverse events were recorded and seroconversion of neutralising antibodies were detected in 92% and 98% of vaccinees receiving doses of 3 and 6 µg, respectively, suggesting the 3 µg dose as being sufficient for a phase III trial. In a phase III study in 18–59-year-old volunteers, the vaccination with two doses of 3 µg was determined safe and the vaccine efficacy was estimated as 83.5% [49]. The Sinovac has been approved in China and in several other countries, including the UK at the end of 2021 (www.blog. wego.com/sinovac-approved-countries/).

In the context of **protein subunit vaccines**, a trimeric full-length SARS-CoV-2 S nanoparticle vaccine combined with Matrix-M1 adjuvant has been subjected to phase I/II clinical trials [64]. In the phase I study, 83 participants received two intramuscular injections of 5 or 25 µg SARS-CoV-2 S NPs (NVX-CoV2373) with adjuvant, 25 individuals were neutraliz with the vaccine candidate only, and 23 received placebo. No serious adverse events were registered. The neutralizing induced Th1 responses and elicited neutralizing antibody responses, which were enhanced by the addition of the adjuvant. The neutralisation responses exceeded those observed in convalescent serum from COVID-19 patients [50]. In a phase III trial on co-administration of NVX-CoV2373 and a seasonal influenza vaccine the safety, immunogenicity, and efficacy were evaluated [51]. Although the safety was acceptable, reactogenicity was more common after co-administration of the two vaccines than for NVX-CoV2373 alone. Moreover, co-administration did not affect the immune response against influenza virus. However, the antibody response against NVX-CoV2373 was reduced. Despite that, the NVX-CoV2373 vaccine efficacy was 87.5–89.8%. In another phase III trial, adults 18–84-years old received two intramuscular doses of 5 µg NVX-CoV2373 [52]. A vaccine efficacy of 89.7% was achieved and no hospitalisation or deaths were recorded among 10 breakthrough infections. Moreover, NVX-CoV2373 showed an 86.3% efficacy against the SARS-CoV-2 B.1.1.7 (alpha) variant and 96.4% against non-B.1.1.7 variants. The NVX-CoV2373 vaccine has received Emergency Use Authorization (EUA) in the EU and the UK [53]. Another protein subunit vaccine ZF2001, based on the SARS-CoV-2 S RBD dimer produced in CHO cells, has been subjected to phase I and phase II trials [54]. In the phase I trial, three doses of 25 or 50 µg of ZF2001 were administered to 50 volunteers and in the phase II trial 900 participants received two or three doses of 25 or 50 µg of ZF2001 intramuscularly. Both doses were well tolerated in the phase I study. In phase II, the seroconversion rates of neutralising antibodies were 72% for the 25 µg dose and 72% for the 50 µg dose after two vaccinations and 97% for 25 µg and 93% for 50 µg after three vaccinations. Overall, 25 µg has been selected for a three-dose regimen in a phase III trial.

Viral vector-based vaccines have seen plenty of progress in clinical trials. Ad-based vectors have been on the forefront with several clinical studies completed or currently in progress. For instance, in a dose-escalation, open-label, non-randomised phase I study 108 healthy 18–60 year-old volunteers received 5×10^{10}, 1×10^{11}, or 1.5×10^{11} Ad5 particles expressing the SARS-CoV-2 S protein (Ad5-nCoV) [55]. No serious adverse events were discovered after vaccination and peak humoral immune responses were detected at 28 days and rapid T-cell responses 14 days after immunisation. The Ad5-nCoV vaccine candidate was subjected to a randomised, double-blind, placebo-controlled phase II study in 603 volunteers receiving either 5×10^{10} or 1×10^{11} Ad particles [56]. No serious adverse reactions were recorded and both doses induced significant neutralising antibody responses in the majority of vaccinees after a single immunisation. In another phase I/II trial, Ad5-nCoV was administered to individuals with and without prior COVID-19 [57]. No vaccine-related adverse events were discovered. Higher neutralising antibodies were detected in individuals with prior COVID-19. For this reason, a booster Ad5-nCoV dose is recommended. In a multi-nation phase III trial, a single dose of 5×10^{10} Ad5-nCoV particles did not cause any significant difference in the incidence of serious adverse events compared to placebo [58]. Moreover, interim results indicated a vaccine efficacy of 57.5%. The Ad5-nCoV vaccine received EUA in ten countries, most being low-income countries, before the final results from phase III studies were available [59]. The main reasons for this were the acute pandemic and the lack of access to approved COVD-19 vaccines. Fortunately, the Ad5-nCoV safety and efficacy were acceptable in providing protection to the millions of people receiving the vaccine. In another approach, the Ad5-nCoV vaccine was subjected to intranasal aerosolised and intramuscular administration in a phase I trial [60]. Intranasal delivery of a low dose (1×10^{10} particles) and high dose (2×10^{10} particles) was followed by the same booster dose after 28 days. Moreover, some individuals received a mixed regimen of intramuscular Ad5-nCoV (5×10^{10} particles) followed by an aerosolised booster of 2×10^{10} on day 28, or one dose of 5×10^{10} or two doses of 10×10^{10} particles intramuscularly. Clearly, the intramuscular route caused more adverse events in comparison to intranasal administration. Two doses of aerosolised Ad5-nCoV generated similar neutralising antibody responses compared to one intramuscular dose. Moreover, intramuscular administration followed by intranasal booster delivery after 28 days induced strong IgG and neutralising antibody responses.

In another approach, the COVID-19 vaccine candidate based on the Ad type 26 vector has been subjected to a randomised, double-blind, placebo-controlled phase I/II clinical trial in 1045 healthy individuals in Belgium and the US [61]. Preliminary results from the phase I/II trial demonstrated that a single immunisation with 5×10^{10} Ad26.COV2.S particles showed a good safety profile and potentially provided protection against COVID-19. In another phase I study, a single immunisation with Ad26.COV2.S elicited rapid binding and neutralisation antibodies in volunteers [62]. In a phase III trial, a single dose of 5×10^{10} Ad26.COV2.S particles protected against moderate to severe-critical COVID-19 with a vaccine efficacy of 66.9% [63]. Moreover, a vaccine efficacy of 85.4% was achieved against severe COVID-19. Ad26.COV2.S was granted EUA in February 2021 by the FDA (www.jnj.com). The approach of prime-boost vaccination with rAd26-S and rAd5-S surprisingly resulted in the premature approval in Russia before any clinical results were published [64]. Eventually, results published from a phase I/II trial demonstrated a good safety profile without any serious adverse reactions and strong SARS-CoV-2-specific antibody responses in all vaccinees [20]. Furthermore, interim results from a phase III study showed a vaccine efficacy of 91.6% [65]. The chimpanzee ChAdOx1–based vaccine candidate has been subjected to a single-blinded, randomised controlled phase I/II study in healthy adults aged 18–55 by a single intramuscular administration of 5×10^{10} ChADOx1 nCoV-19 viral particles [66]. Overall, 1,077 patients were enrolled in the study. Preliminary observations showed no serious adverse events related to ChAdOx1 nCoV-19 [66]. Neutralising antibody responses against SARS-CoV-2 were detected in 32 (91%) of 35 participants after a single dose, which rose to 100% after a booster dose. Moreover, more frequent adverse events were registered in younger individuals in a phase II/III trial [67]. In contrast, there was no difference in neutralising antibody titres in individuals 18–55 years, 56–69 years, and 70 years and older. Interim results from a phase III trial in the UK, Brazil, and South Africa showed good safety and provided 62.1% vaccine efficacy after immunisation with two doses of 5×10^{10} ChAdOx1 nCoV-19 [68]. Furthermore, vaccination with a prime dose of 2.2×10^{10} particles and a boost dose of 5.5×10^{10} particles of ChAdOx1 nCoV-19 provided 90% vaccine efficacy. EUA was granted for ChAdOx1 nCoV-19 in the UK in December 2020 [69].

COVID-19 **DNA vaccine** candidates have also been subjected to clinical trials. In this context, the INO-4800 vaccine candidate based on the pGX9501 DNA plasmid expressing the full-length SARS-CoV-2 S protein was administered intradermally in combination with electroporation to 120 healthy volunteers aged 18 years and older in a phase I study in the United States [70]. The study showed excellent safety and tolerability profiles. Immunogenicity was achieved in all 38 vaccinated volunteers, eliciting either humoral or cellular immune responses, or both. In another phase I trial, two doses of 0.5, 1.0, and 2.0 mg of the INO-4800 vaccine were administered intradermally followed by electroporation at four weeks intervals including an optional booster vaccination 6–10 months later [71]. The treatment was well tolerated with no serious adverse events recorded. The antibody response was durable, and it was significantly enhanced by booster immunisation. Moreover, a phase II/III study was conducted on safety, immunogenicity, and efficacy of the INO-4800 in more than 7,000 individuals (NCT04642638). Another DNA-based vaccine candidate (AG0301-COVID-19) expressing multiple SARS-CoV-2 specific antigens has been subjected to two phase I/II clinical trials. Approximately 30 healthy volunteers have been enrolled in one phase I/II study, where one half of them are subjected to intramuscular administration of a low dose of 1.0 mg DNA and the other half to a high dose of 2.0 mg DNA (NCT04463472). In the other study, a single-center, randomised, open-label, non-controlled phase I/II trial in 30 healthy volunteers will be subjected to two intramuscular administrations twice at two-week intervals, twice at four-week intervals, and three times at two-week intervals, respectively (NCT04527081). The Indian plasmid DNA–based SARS-CoV-2 S vaccine (ZyCoV-D) has been subjected to a phase I trial, where three doses were administered at 28 day intervals [72]. Out of 48 vaccinated individuals, at least one adverse event was detected in 12 subjects. Overall, ZyCoV-D was safe, well tolerated, and elicited strong immune responses. In a phase III trial, in more than 27,000 participants receiving three doses of ZyCoV-D the number of adverse events was similar to those seen for the placebo group and showed a vaccine efficacy of 66.6% [73]. ZyCoV-D was approved in September 2021 in India [74]. Phase I trials have also been conducted with the plasmid DNA–based GX-19 and GX-19N vaccine candidates in South Korea [75]. The former contains the SARS-CoV-2 S gene and the latter both the SARS-CoV-2 S and N genes. Only mild adverse events except for one case of moderate fatigue were recorded in vaccinated healthy adults aged 19–54 years. Robust binding antibody responses were detected for both vaccine candidates, which were enhanced after the second dose.

RNA–based vaccines represent the most innovative and novel approach for vaccine development against COVID-19. In this context, a randomised, double-blind, placebo-controlled phase I/II trial in healthy adult volunteers was conducted by intramuscular administration of the ARCT-021 vaccine candidate, the lipid-based LUNAR® multi-component delivery system for SARS-CoV-2 mRNA [76]. In phase I, safety, tolerability, and immunogenicity were evaluated after a single ascending dose of ARCT-021, showing good tolerance up to a dose of 7.5 μg. The phase II comprised two doses of 5.0 μg of ARCT-021 administered 28 days apart. Adverse events included injection site pain, fatigue, headache, and myalgia. The seroconversion rate of anti-S IgG was 100% and the titers comparable to those found in convalescent COVID-19 patients. In another RNA–based vaccine development approach, the thermostable LNP encapsulated mRNA for SARS-CoV-2 S RBD (ARCoV) [77] has been subjected to clinical trials in China. In a phase I study, two immunisations with doses of 5, 10, 15, 20, and 25 μg ARCoV mRNA was administered to healthy 18–59 year-old volunteers [78]. Only mild or moderate adverse events were recorded, fever being the most common adverse reaction. The vaccination elicited humoral responses against the SARS-CoV-2 S RBD and neutralising antibodies, which showed significantly higher titres after the second immunisation. The highest neutralising antibodies were obtained with the 15 μg dose, which was two times higher compared to the antibody titers measured from convalescent COVID-19 patients. Another mRNA-based vaccine, CVnCoV, encoding the SARS-CoV-2 S protein has been subjected to a partially blind, placebo-controlled, dose-escalation phase I clinical trial for the evaluation of safety and immunogenicity in 245 healthy adults [79]. The study demonstrated that there were no vaccine-related serious adverse events. Moreover, dose-dependent increase in IgG antibodies against SARS-CoV-2 S and RBD was observed. It was determined that 12 μg of CVnCoV mRNA overlapped immune responses from convalescent COVID-19 patients.

Several clinical trials have been conducted for the BNT162b1/b2 mRNA vaccine candidates. For example, in a phase I/II study, the BNT162b1 vaccine the evaluation of safety, tolerability, and immunogenicity demonstrated a dose-dependent, generally mild to moderate presence of local and systemic adverse events [80]. The neutralising antibody titers were 1.9 to 4.6-fold higher than detected in the sera of convalescent COVID-19 patients. In a phase I dose-escalation trial, both BNT162b1 and BNT162b2 showed similar or higher SARS-CoV-2 neutralising titres compared to those of convalescent COVID-19 patients [81]. However, BNT162b2 showed a lower incidence of severe adverse events than BNT162b1, especially in older individuals. Furthermore, the BNT162b2 vaccine candidate showed a 95% vaccine efficacy in a phase III study in 43,548 individuals [82]. The BNT162b2 vaccine was granted EUA in the UK, Europe, and the US in late 2020 and early 2021 [83]. The LNP-mRNA-1273 vaccine candidate has also been subjected to several clinical trials. For example, two intramuscular injections of doses ranging from 10 to 250 μg of LNP-mRNA-1273 were administered to 150 volunteers in a phase I trial [84]. Anti-SARS-CoV-2 immune responses were observed in all participants. The antibody responses correlated with increased dose and the antibody titres were significantly higher after the second dose. Preliminary results from a phase II trial caused only mild severe adverse reactions such as pain at the injection site, headache, and fatigue [85]. Both binding and neutralising antibodies were detected, again at substantially increased levels after the second vaccination, which exceeded the levels seen in COVID-19 patients. Moreover, in a phase III study in 30,420 volunteers, the LNP-mRNA-1273 vaccine efficacy was estimated as 94.1% [86]. The LNP-mRNA-1273 vaccine was granted approval in the US in December 2020 [87]. In a first-in-human, randomised, placebo-controlled, observer-blind, dose-finding phase I study for the LNP-saRNA–based vaccine candidate LNP-nCoVsaRNA [88], six doses of 0-1-10 µg were well tolerated and elicited immune responses at relatively modest levels, failing to induce 100% seroconversion.

COVID-19 Vaccines and Cancer Patients

One issue of importance related to mass vaccinations against SARS-CoV-2 has been to assess the safety and immunogenicity of the newly engineered COVID-19 vaccines in cancer patients [89]. In a phase I trial, patients with solid tumors and haematological cancer were subjected to intramuscular administration of the BNT162b2 vaccine and compared to healthy volunteers [89]. Positive anti-S IgG titres were detected in 32 out of 34 healthy controls (94%), in 21 out of 56 patients with solid tumors (38%), and in 8 out of 44 individuals with haematological cancer (18%). After the second immunisation, 12 out of 12 healthy controls (100%), 18 out 19 patients with solid tumors (95%), and 3 out of 5 patients with haematological cancer (60%) were sero-positive. The study showed that the vaccination was safe, and the relatively poor vaccine efficacy in patients with solid cancer could be significantly improved by a second vaccination. In a phase III trial, the BNT162b2 vaccine was administered to patients with breast and prostate cancer, and melanoma in comparison to placebo [90]. Among patients vaccinated with BNT162b2, four patients developed COVID-19 compared to 71 individuals receiving placebo, indicating a vaccine efficacy of 95%. It compared favorably with an overall vaccine efficacy of 91.1%. The cancer patients tolerated the vaccination well with only mild adverse reactions such as injection-site pain, fatigue, and pyrexia. Overall, the safety and efficacy profiles were similar to those seen in the general population. Application of COVID-19 vaccines has raised some concern about the immune alterations related to cancers or cancer therapy [91].

The presence of spike-reactive or RBD–reactive antibodies have been detected in cancer patients, eliciting neutralising antibodies also against variants of concern (VoC) in some cases [92–97]. Only in a few studies have T-cell responses been induced and often in smaller subsets, and therefore additional research is needed to validate the observed effects. Different studies reported that cancer patients developed a less proficient immune response after vaccination against COVID-19 compared with healthy individuals without cancer [89, 98–104]. In addition, a 75% efficacy of mRNA vaccines against COVID-19 hospitalisation in cancer patients was calculated before the Omicron variant became predominant [105]. Moreover, it was found that elderly people showed vaccine efficacy (VE). In the same study the VE was reduced due to the high prevalence of the Delta variant [105]. In another study conducted only in cancer patients, the VE was estimated at approximately 60% [106]. Naturally, VE was correlated with timing of cancer therapy, and it ranged from 54% in patients receiving any therapy (including endocrine therapies, targeted therapies, and/or chemotherapy) to 85% in those not treated within the past 6 months. A cohort study involving almost seven million vaccinated participants in the UK found different risk factors for COVID-19–related death despite vaccination with two doses: patients who received moderate-to-high intensity chemotherapy, or stem cell transplantation within the past 6 months; patients with haematological cancer; and terminal patients with respiratory tract cancer [107]. In this regard, patients with haematological malignancies are most likely to be affected. Specifically, 56% of these patients elicited detectable neutralising antibody titres against the ancestral Wuhan strain, whereas only 31% showed detectable titres against the Delta variant after two vaccine doses [92]. Initial results indicated that neutralising antibodies against Omicron increased from 47.8% to 88.9% after a third vaccine dose in patients with solid tumors [108]. Specifically, patients with non-small-cell lung cancer showed a 79-fold lower neutralising antibody titre to Omicron than individuals without cancer after two doses of an mRNA vaccine [109]. In patients with haematological malignancies, neutralising antibodies against Omicron were rarely detected after two vaccine doses, although approximately 50% showed detectable neutralising antibodies after a third dose [110]. In another study, patients with solid tumors showed comparable [92, 93, 111] or reduced [102, 104, 112] antibody titres to healthy individuals after two vaccine doses. A meta-analysis of data derived from four studies on fully vaccinated patients with solid tumors [103] reported a reduced antibody titre in comparison to individuals without cancer. Differences in seroconversion between patients with solid tumours and healthy individuals are probably moderate and/or restricted to specific subgroups. In many cases, chemotherapy (received from within 28 days to 6 months of vaccination) has been identified as a risk factor for low seroconversion and neutralising antibodies, although not in all studies [92, 108]. Furthermore, 46–79% of patients with solid tumors showed detectable T-cell responses after vaccination against COVID-19, considering IFNγ release [92, 93, 113], combined IFNγ and IL-2 release [106, 108], or flow cytometric analysis of cellular activation-induced markers [114]. In addition, cancer patients showed discordant antibody and cellular responses [92, 96, 106, 108]. In this regard, it is very difficult to determine risk factors for poor T-cell responses to vaccination. Several factors have been indicated: firstly, differences between applied assays can influence the observed responses, and no unified cut-off for positive T-cell responses exists. Secondly, T-cell responses have often been observed in subsets of patients, such as those with no seroconversion, thereby limiting the ability to detect less overt risk factors. Nevertheless, patients who have received treatment for cancer [106, 114] such as chemotherapy [96], steroids, or immune checkpoint inhibitors within 15 days of vaccination [96] showed reduced T-cell responses to vaccination. In addition, T cells can be detected also in the absence of antibody responses in these patients [96]. Moreover, T-cell responses against spike peptide pools specific for VoC have also been found [92]. In a study in Turkey, 64% of a total of 47 patients with solid tumours, who mostly received chemotherapy or immune checkpoint inhibitors after vaccination with the inactivated CoronaVac virus vaccine, showed seroconversion [115]. In another study in Iran, 87% of a total of 364 cancer patients showed serological responses after two doses of the BBIBP-CorV vaccine [116]. Several studies have shown that patients with haematological malignancies elicited low immune responses after COVID-19 vaccinations [92, 95, 105, 106, 111, 113, 117] and also showed a lower VE in a large-cohort study in the US [107]. Encouragingly long-term survivors of haematological malignancies, including stem cell transplant recipients, show a similar response to vaccination as seen in the general population, even in the case of prior therapy being very immunosuppressive [108, 118]. However, it has been documented that certain anticancer therapies can reduce humoral immune response to vaccination, especially for all B-cell–depleting treatments (including CD20, BCMA, and CD38–targeted therapies). Furthermore, the spike protein-reactive IgG responses can be associated with the absolute number of B cells in patients [119]. For this reason, the suppressive effects of B-cell–depleting therapies can last for ≥1 year after treatment cessation [111, 120], putting these patients at an increased risk of breakthrough infections.

Furthermore, some studies reported robust T-cell responses, with 30–75% of seronegative patients having specific T-cell responses to vaccination independent of disease subtype [92, 113, 121, 122]. Patients with haematological malignancies often show discordant humoral and cellular responses to vaccination compared with other populations [114]. Furthermore, the patients subjected to ongoing treatment with B-cell–depleting therapies showed T-cell responses to vaccination [121], highlighting that the ability of these patients to develop adaptive immunity is not completely disrupted. Moreover, T-cell responses, most importantly CD8+ responses, have been found in cancer patients receiving B-cell–depleting therapies who subsequently developed COVID-19, even in the absence of humoral responses [123–125], indicating that T-cell responses alone can provide protection from severe outcomes.

Conclusions and Future Aspects

The efforts to develop vaccines against COVID-19 in response to the global pandemic has been unprecedented. Encouraging news has been reported for two RNA–based vaccines from Pfizer/BioNTech and Moderna, respectively. In both cases LNP formulations for modified mRNA have been applied, which has generated over 90% vaccine efficacy in phase III trials. Moreover, Ad-based ChAdOx1 nCoV-2 vaccine and the single-dose Ad26.COV2.S vaccine have demonstrated promising efficacy results in phase III clinical trials. All four vaccines have been granted EUA in various countries around the globe. Additionally, the protein-based NVX-CoV2373 has also received EUA in Europe and the UK. However, the emergence of SARS-CoV-2 mutants/variants has sincerely affected the vaccine efficacy requiring additional booster vaccinations and re-engineering of vaccines.

Importantly, as mass vaccinations have taken place globally, one important question concerns the fate of cancer patients. Results from several clinical trials have indicated that vaccination of cancer patients is safe, and although relatively inferior immune responses compared to healthy individuals have been recorded, booster immunisations have provided improved immunogenicity. Overall, it seems that the benefits of subjecting cancer patients to vaccination outweighs the risks of severe adverse effects and the severity of COVID-19.

REFERENCES

1. Zhao L, Jha BK, Wu A, et al. Antagonism of the interferon-induced OAS-RNase L pathway by murine coronavirus ns2 protein is required for virus replication and liver pathology. *Cell Host Microbe* 2012;11:607–616. doi: 10.1016/j.chom.2012.04.011.
2. Ou X, Liu Y, Lei X, et al. Characterization of spike glycoprotein of SARS-CoV-2 on virus entry and its immune cross-reactivity with SARS-CoV. *Nat Commun* 2020;11:1620. https://doi.org/10.1038/s41467-020-15562-9.

3. Sarkar M, Saha S. Structural insight into the role of novel SARS-CoV-2 E protein: A potential target for vaccine development and other therapeutic strategies. *PLOS ONE* 2020;15(8):e0237300. doi: 10.1371/journal.pone.0237300.

4. Ribet D, Cossart P. How bacterial pathogens colonize their hosts and invade deeper tissues. *Microbes Infect* 2015;17:173–183. doi: 10.1016/j.micinf.2015.01.004.

5. Wang H, Zhang Y, Huang B, et al. Development of an inactivated vaccine candidate, BBIBP-CorV, with potent protection against SARS-CoV-2. *Cell* 2020;182:713–721. https://doi.org/10.1016/j.cell.2020.06.008.

6. Gao Q, Bao L, Mao H, et al. Development of an inactivated vaccine candidate for SARS-CoV-2. *Science* 2020;369:77–81. doi:10.1126/science.abc1932.

7. Cheng BYH, Ortiz-Riano E, Nogales A, et al. Development of live-attenuated arenavirus vaccines based on codon deoptimization. *J Virol* 2015;89:3523–3533. doi: 10.1128/JVI.03401-14.

8. Li T, Zheng Q, Yu H, et al. SARS-CoV-2 spike produced in insect cells elicits high neutralization titers in non-human primates. *Emerg Microbes Infect* 2020; 9:2076–2090. doi: 10.1080/22221751.2020.1821583.

9. An X, Martinez-Paniagua M, Rezvan A, et al. Single-dose intranasal vaccination elicits systemic and mucosal immunity against SARS-CoV-2. *iScience* 2021 Sep 24;24(9):103037. doi: 10.1016/j.isci.2021.103037.

10. Battacharaya M, Sharma AR, Patra P, et al . Development of epitope-based vaccine against novel coronavirus 2019 (SARS-CoV-2): Immunoinformatics approach. *J Med Virol* 2020;92:618–631. doi: 10.1002/jmv.25736.

11. Lin L, Ting S, Yufei H, et al. Epitope-based peptide vaccines predicted against novel coronavirus disease caused by SARS-CoV-2. *Virus Res* 2020;288:198082. doi: 10.1016/j.virusres.2020.198082.

12. Kalita P, Padhi AK, Zhang KYJ, et al. Design of a peptide-based subunit vaccine against novel coronavirus SARS-CoV-2. *Microb Pathog* 2020;145:104236. doi: 10.1016/j.micpath.2020.104236.

13. Baig MS, Alagumuthu M, Rajpoot S, et al. Identification of a potential peptide inhibitor of SARS-COv-2 targeting its entry into host cells. *Drugs R D* 2020;20:161–169. doi: 10.1007/s40268-020-00312-5.

14. Lundstrom K. Viral vector-based vaccines against COVID-19. *Explor Immunol* 2022;1:295–308. doi: 10.37349/ei.2021.00020.

15. Folegatti PM, Bellamy D, Roberts R, et al. Safety and immunogenicity of a novel recombinant simian Adenovirus ChAdOx2 as a vectored vaccine. *Vaccines* 2019;7:40. doi: 10.3390/vaccines7020040.

16. van Doremalen N, Lambe T, Spencer A, et al. ChAdOx1 nCov-19 vaccination prevents SARS-CoV-2 pneumonia in rhesus macaques. *Nature* 2020;586:578–582. doi: 10.1038/s41586-020-2608-y.

17. Feng L, Wang Q, Shan C, et al. An adenovirus-vectored COVID-19 vaccine confers protection from SARS-CoV-2 challenge in rhesus macaques. *Nat Commun* 2020;11:4207. doi: 10.1038/s41467-020-18077-5.

18. Tostanoski LH, Wegmann F, Martinot AJ, et al. Ad26 vaccine protects against SARS-CoV-2 severe clinical disease in hamsters. *Nat Med Nat Med* 2020;26(11):1694–1700. doi: 10.1038/s41591-020-1070-6.

19. Mercado NNB, Zahn R, Wegmann F, et al. Single-shot Ad26 vaccine protects against SARS-CoV-2 in rhesus macaques. *Nature* 2020;586:583–588. doi: 10.1038/s41586-020-2607-z.

20. Logunov DY, Dolzhikova IV, Zubkova OV, et al. Safety and immunogenicity of an rAd26 and rAd5 vector-based heterologous prime-boost COVID-19 vaccine in two

formulations: Two open, non-randomised phase 1/2 studies from Russia. *Lancet* 2020;396:887–897. doi: 10.1016/S0140-6736(20)31866-3.

21. Lee J, Kumar SA, Jhan YY, et al. Engineering DNA vaccines against infectious diseases. *Acta Biomater* 2018;80:31–47. doi: 10.1016/j.actbio.2018.08.033.

22. Wolff JA, Malone RW, Williams P, et al. Direct gene transfer into mouse muscle in vivo, *Science* 1990;247(4949):1465–1468. doi: 10.1126/science.1690918.

23. Hooper JW, Moon JE, Paolino KM, et al. A phase 1 clinical trial of Hantaan virus and Puumala virus M-segment DNA vaccines for haemorrhagic fever with renal syndrome delivered by intramuscular electroporation. *Clin Microbiol Infect* 2014;20:110–117. doi: 10.1111/1469-0691.12553.

24. McBurney SP, Sunshine JE, Gabriel S, et al. (2016). Evaluation of protection induced by a dengue virus serotype 2 envelope domain III protein scaffold/DNA vaccine in non-human primates. *Vaccine* 34:3500–3507. doi: 10.1016/j.vaccine.2016.03.108.

25. Lundstrom K, Boulikas T. Viral and non-viral vectors in gene therapy: Technology development and clinical trials. *Technol Cancer Res Treat* 2003;2:471–486. doi: 10.1177/153303460300200513.

26. Sunshine JC, Bishop CJ, Green JJ. Advances in polymeric and inorganic vectors for nonviral nucleic acid delivery. *Ther Deliv* 2011;2:493–521. doi: 10.4155/tde.11.14.

27. Darquet AM, Cameron B, Wils P, et al. A new DNA vehicle for nonviral gene delivery: Supercoiled minicircle. *Gene Ther* 1997;4:1341–1349. doi: 10.1038/sj.gt.3300540.

28. Huang M, Chen Z, Hu S, et al. Novel minicircle vector for gene therapy in murine myocardial infarction. *Circulation* 2009;120:S230–S237. doi:10.1161/CIRCULATIONAHA.108.841155.

29. Shen X, Pitol AK, Bachmann V, et al. A simple plasmid-based transient gene expression method using high five cells. *J Biotechnol* 2015;216:67–75. doi: 10.1016/j.jbiotec.2015.10.007.

30. Sun J, Li D, Hao Y, et al. Posttranscriptional regulatory elements enhance antigen expression and DNA vaccine efficacy. *DNA Cell Biol* 2009;28, 233–240. doi: 10.1089/dna.2009.0862.

31. Grantham R, Gautier C, Gouy M, et al. Codon catalog usage and the genome hypothesis. *Nucl Acids Res* 1980;8:r49–r62. doi: 10.1093/nar/8.1.197-c.

32. Smith TRF, Patel A, Ramos S, et al. Immunogenicity of a DNA vaccine candidate for COVID-19. *Nat Commun* 2020;11:2601. doi: 10.1038/s41467-020-16505.

33. Yu J, Tostanoski LH, Peter L, et al. DNA vaccine protection against SARS-CoV-2 in rhesus macaques. *Science* 2020;369:806–811. doi: 10.1126/science.abc6284.

34. Stepinski J Waddell C, Stolarski R, et al. Synthesis and properties of mRNAs containing the novel 'anti-reverse' cap analogs 7-methyl (3'-*O*-methyl) GpppG and 7-methyl (33'-deoxy) GpppG, *RNA* 2001;7:1486–1495.

35. Munroe D, Jacobson A. mRNA poly(A) tail, a 3' enhancer of translational initiation. *Mol Cell Biol* 1990;10:3441–3455. doi: 10.1128/mcb.10.7.3441.

36. Kariko K, Muramatsu H, Welsh FA, et al. Incorporation of pseudouridine into mRNA yields superior nonimmunogenic vector with increased translational capacity and biological stability. *Mol Ther* 2008;16:1833–1840. doi: 10.1038/mt.2008.200.

37. Wang Y, Li Z, Han Y, et al. Nanoparticle-based delivery system for application of siRNA in vivo. *Curr Drug Metab* 2010;11:182–196. doi: 10.2174/138920010791110863.

38. Lundstrom, K. Latest development on RNA-based drugs and vaccines. *Future Sci OA* 2018;4:FSO300. doi: 10.4155/fsoa-2017-0151.

39. Blakney AK, McKay PF, Yus BI, et al. Inside out: Optimization of lipid nanoparticle formulations for exterior complexation and in vivo delivery of saRNA. *Gene Ther* 2019;26:363–372. doi: 10.1038/s41434-019-0095-2.

40. Corbett KS, Edwards DK, Leist SR, et al. SARS-CoV-2 mRNA vaccine design enabled by prototype pathogen preparedness. *Nature* 2020;586:567–571. https://doi.org/10.1038/s41586-020-2622-0.

41. Corbett KS, Flynn B, Foulds KE, et al. Evaluation of the mRNA-1273 vaccine against SARS-CoV-2 in nonhuman primates. *N Engl J Med* 2020;383:1544–1555. doi: 10.1056/NEJMoa2024671.

42. Vogel AB, Kanevsky I, Che Y, et al. BNT162b vaccines protect rhesus macaques from SARS-CoV-2. *Nature* 2021;592:283–289. doi: 10.1038/s41586-021-03275-y.

43. https://www.curevac.com/covid-19 (cited September 26, 2022).

44. https://arcturusrx.com (cited September 26, 2022).

45. Zhang B, Chao CW, Tsybovsky Y, et al. A platform incorporating trimeric antigens into self-assembling nanoparticles reveals SARS-CoV-2-spike nanoparticles to elicit substantially higher neutralizing antibodies than spike alone. *Sci Rep* 2020;10:18149. doi: 10.1038/s41598-020-74949-2.

46. Xia S, Duan K, Zhang Y, et al Effect of an inactivated vaccine against SARS-CoV-2 on safety and immunogenicity outcomes. Interim analysis of 2 randomized clinical trials. *JAMA* 2020;324(10):951–960. doi: 10.1001/jama.2020.15543.

47. Xia S, Zhang Y, Wang Y, et al. Safety and immunogenicity of an inactivated SARS-CoV-2 vaccine, BBIBP-CorV: A randomised, double-blind, placebo-controlled, phase 1/2 trial. *Lancet Infect Dis* 2021;21(1):39–51. doi: 10.1016/S1473-3099(20)30831-8.

48. Zhang Y, Zeng G, Pan H, et al. Safety, tolerability and immunogenicity of an inactivated SARS-CoV-2 vaccine in healthy adults aged 18–59 years: A randomised, double-blind, placebo-controlled, phase 1/2 clinical trial. *Lancet Infect Dis* 2021;21(2):181–192. https://doi.org/10.1016/S1473-3099(20)30870-7.

49. Tanriover MD, Doğanay HL, Akova M, et al. Efficacy and safety of an inactivated whole-virion SARS-CoV-2 vaccine (CoronaVac): Interim results of a double-blind, randomised, placebo-controlled, phase 3 trial in Turkey. *Lancet* 2021;398:213–222. doi: 10.1016/S0140-6736(21)01429-X.

50. Keech C, Albert G, Cho I, et al. Phase 1–2 trial of a SARS-CoV-2 recombinant spike protein nanoparticle vaccine. *N Engl J Med* 2020;383(24):2320–2332. doi: 10.1056/NEJMoa2026920.

51. Toback S, Galiza E, Cosgrove C, et al. Safety, immunogenicity, and efficacy of a COVID-19 vaccine (NVX-CoV2373) co-administered with seasonal influenza vaccines: An exploratory substudy of a randomised, observer-blinded, placebo-controlled, phase 3 trial. *Lancet Respir Med* 2022;10:167–179. doi: 10.1016/S2213-2600(21)00409-4.

52. Heath PT, Galiza EP, Baxter DN et al safety and efficacy of NVX-CoV2373 Covid-19 vaccine. *N Engl J Med* 2021;385:1172–1183. doi: 10.1056/NEJMoa2107659.

53. Parums DV. Editorial: First approval of the protein-based adjuvanted nuvaxovid (NVX-CoV2373) novavax vaccine for SARS-CoV-2 could increase vaccine uptake and provide immune protection from viral variants. *Med Sci Monit* 2022;28:e936523. doi: 10.12659/MSM.936523.

54. Yang S, Li Y, Dai L, et al. Safety and immunogenicity of a recombinant tandem-repeat dimeric RBD-based protein subunit vaccine (ZF2001) against COVID-19 in adults: Two randomised, double-blind, placebo-controlled, phase 1 and 2 trials. *Lancet Infect Dis* 2021;21:1107–1119. doi: 10.1016/S1473-3099(21)00127-4.

55. Zhu F-C, Li Y-H, Guan X-H, et al. Safety, tolerability, and immunogenicity of a recombinant adenovirus type-5 vectored COVID-19 vaccine: A dose-escalation,

open-label, non-randomised, first-in-human trial. *Lancet* 2020;395:1845–1854. doi: 10.1016/S0140-6736(20)31208-3.

56. Zhu F-C, Guan X-H, Li Y-H, et al. Immunogenicity and safety of adenovirus type-5-vectored COVID-19 vaccine in healthy adults ages 18 years or older: A randomised, double-blind, placebo-controlled, phase II trial. *Lancet* 2020;396:479–488. doi: 10.1016/S0140-6736(20)31605-6.

57. Hernández-Bello J, Morales-Núñez JJ, Machado-Sulbarán AC, et al. Neutralizing antibodies against SARS-CoV-2, anti-Ad5 antibodies, and reactogenicity in response to Ad5-nCoV (CanSino biologics) vaccine in individuals with and without prior SARS-CoV-2. *Vaccines* 2021;9:1047. doi: 10.3390/vaccines9091047.

58. Halperin SA, Ye L, MacKinnon-Cameron D, et al. Final efficacy analysis, interim safety analysis, and immunogenicity of a single dose of recombinant novel coronavirus vaccine (adenovirus type 5 vector) in adults 18 years and older: An international, multicentre, randomised, double-blinded, placebo-controlled phase 3 trial. *Lancet* 2022;399:237–248. doi: 10.1016/S0140-6736(21)02753-7.

59. Nunez I. Vaccine approval before phase 3 trial results: A consequence of vaccine access inequity. *Lancet* 2022;399:1223–1224. https://doi.org/10.1016/S0140-6736(2)00164-7.

60. Wu S, Huang J, Zhang Z, et al (2021). Safety, tolerability, and immunogenicity of an aerosolised adenovirus type-5 vector-based COVID-19 vaccine (Ad5-nCoV) in adults: Preliminary report of an open-label and randomised phase 1 clinical trial. *Lancet Infect Dis* 21:1654–1664. doi: 10.1016/S1473-3099(21)00396-0.

61. Sadoff J, Le Gars M, Shukarev G, et al. Interim results of a phase 1–2 a trial of Ad26.COV2.S Covid-19 vaccine. *N Engl J Med* 2021;384:1824–1835. doi: 10.1056/NEJMoa2034201.

62. Stephenson KE, Le Gars M, Sadoff J, et al. Immunogenicity of the Ad26.COV2.S vaccine for COVID-19. *JAMA* 2021;325:1535–1544. doi: 10.1001/jama.2021.3645.

63. Sadoff J, Gray G, Vandebosch A, et al. Safety and efficacy of single-dose Ad26.COV2.S vaccine against Covid-19. *N Engl J Med* 384:2187–2201. doi: 10.1056/NEJMoa2101544.

64. Callaway E. Russia's fast-track coronavirus vaccine draws outrage over safety. *Nature* 2020;584:334–335. doi: 10.1038/d41586-020-02386-2.

65. Logunov DY, Dolzhikova IV, Shcheblyakov DV, et al. Safety and efficacy of an rAd26 and rAd5 vector-based heterologous prime-boost COVID-19: An interim analysis of a randomised controlled phase 3 in Russia. *Lancet* 2021;397:671–681. doi: 10.1016/S0140-6736(21)00234-8.

66. Folegatti PM, Ewer KJ, Aley PK, et al. Safety and immunogenicity of the ChAdOx1 nCoV-19 vaccine against SARS-CoV-2: A preliminary report of a phase 1/2, single-blind, randomized controlled trial. *Lancet* 2020;396:467–478. doi: 10.1016/S0140-6736(20)31604-4.

67. Ramasamy MN, Minassian AM, Ewer KJ, et al. Safety and immunogenicity of ChAdOx1 nCoV-19 vaccine administered in a prime-boost regimen in young and old adults (COV002): A single-blind, randomised, controlled, phase 2/3 trial. *Lancet* 2021;396:1979–1993. doi: 10.1016/S0140-6736(20)32466-1.

68. Voysey M, Costa Clemens SA, Madhi SA, et al. Safety and efficacy of the ChAdOx1 nCoV-19 vaccine (AZD1222) against SARS-CoV-2: An interim analysis of four randomised controlled trials in Brazil, South Africa, and the UK. *Lancet* 2021;397:99–111. doi: 10.1016/S0140-6736(20)32661-1.

69. Riad A, Pokorna A, Mekhemar M, et al. Safety of ChAdOx1 nCoV-19 vaccine: Independent evidence from two EU states. *Vaccines* 2021;9:673. https://doi.org/10.3990/vaccines9060673.

70. Tebas P, Yang S, Boyer JD, et al. Safety and immunogenicity of INO-4800 DNA vaccine against SARS-CoV-2: A preliminary report of an open-label, *Phase I clinical trial eClincalMedicine* 2020;31, 100689. https://doi.org/10.1016/j.eclinm.2020.100689.

71. Kraynyak KA, Blackwood E, Agnes J, et al. SARS-CoV-2 DNA vaccine INO-4800 induces durable immune responses capable of being boosted in a phase 1 open-label trial. *J Infect Dis* 2022;225(11):1923–1932. doi: 10.1093/infdis/jiac016.

72. Momin T, Kansagra K, Patel H, et al. Safety and immunogenicity of a DNA SARS-CoV-2 vaccine (ZyCoV-D): Results of an open-label, non-randomized phase I part of phase I/II clinical study by intradermal route in healthy subjects in India. *EClinicalMedicine* 2021;38:101020. doi: 10.1016/j.eclinm.2021.101020.

73. Khobragade A, Bhate S, Ramaiah V, et al. Efficacy, safety, and immunogenicity of the DNA SARS-CoV-2 vaccine (ZyCoV-D): The interim efficacy results of a phase 3, randomised, double-blind, placebo-controlled study in India. *Lancet* 2022;399:1313–1321. doi: 10.1016/S0140-6736(22)00151-9.

74. Mallapaty S. India's DNA COVID vaccine is the first – more are coming. *Nature* 2021;597:161–162. doi: 10.1038/d41586-021-02385-x.

75. Ahn JY, Lee J, Suh YS, et al. Safety and immunogenicity of two recombinant DNA COVID-19 vaccines containing the coding regions of the spike or spike and nucleocapsid proteins: An interim analysis of two open-label, non-randomised, phase I trials in healthy adults. *Lancet Microbe* 2022;3:e173–e183. doi: 10.1016/S2666-5247(21)00358-X.

76. Low JG, de Alwis R, Chen S (2021). A phase I/II randomized, double-blinded, placebo-controlled trial of a self-amplifying COVID-19 mRNA vaccine. *NPJ Vaccines* 2022 Dec 13; 7(1):161. doi: 10.1038/s41541-022-00590-x.

77. Zhang NN, Li XF, Deng YQ, et al. A thermostable mRNA vaccine against COVID-19. *Cell* 2020;182:1271–1283. doi: 10.1016/j.cell.2020.07.024.

78. Chen GL, Li XF, Dai XH, et al. Safety and immunogenicity of the SARS-CoV-2 ARCoV mRNA vaccine in Chinese adults: A randomised, double-blind, placebo-controlled, phase 1 trial. *Lancet Microbe* 2022;3:e193–e202. doi: 10.1016/S2666-5247(21)00280-9.

79. Kremsner PG, Mann P, Kroidl A, et al. Safety and immunogenicity of an mRNA-lipid nanoparticle vaccine candidate against SARS-CoV-2: A phase 1 randomized clinical trial. *Wien Klin Wochenschr* 2021;133:931–941. doi: 10.1007/s00508-021-01922-y.

80. Mulligan MJ, Lyke KE, Kitchin N, et al. Phase I/II study of COVID-19 RNA vaccine BNT162b1 in adults. *Nature* 2020;586:589–593. https://doi.org/10.1038/s41586-020-2639-4.

81. Walsh EE, Frenck RW, Falsey AN, et al. Safety and immunogenicity of two RNA-based COVID-19 vaccine candidates. *N Engl J Med* 2020;NEJMoa2027906. doi: 10.1056/NEJMoa2027906.

82. Polack FP, Thomas SJ, Kitchin N, et al. Safety and efficacy of the BNT162b2 mRNA COVID-19 vaccine. *N Engl J Med* 2020;383:2603–2615. Doi: 10.1056/NEJMoa2034577.

83. Lamb YN. BNT162b2 mRNA COVID-19 vaccine: First approval. *Drugs* 2021;81:495–501. doi: 10.1007/s40265-021-01480-7.

84. Jackson LA, Anderson EJ, Rouphael N, et al. An mRNA vaccine against SARS-CoV-2 – preliminary report. *N Engl J Med* 2020;383:1920–1931. doi: 10.1056/NEJMoa2022483.

85. Chu L, McPhee R, Huang W, et al. A preliminary report of a randomized controlled phase 2 trial of the safety and immunogenicity of mRNA-1273 SARS-CoV-2 vaccine. *Vaccine* 2021;39:2791–2799. doi: 10.1016/j.vaccine.2021.02.007.

86. Baden LR, El Sahly HM, Essink B, et al. Efficacy and safety of the mRNA-1273 SARS-CoV-2 vaccine. *N Engl J Med* 2021;384:403–416. doi: 10.1056/NEJMoa2035389.

87. Oliver SE, Gargano JW, Marin M, et al. The advisory committee on immunization practices' interim recommendation for use of Moderna COVID-19 vaccine – United States, December 2020. *MMWR Morb Mortal Wkly Rep* 2021;69:1653–1656. doi: 10.15585/mmwr.mm695152e1.

88. Pollock KM, Cheeseman HM, Szubert AJ, et al. Safety and immunogenicity of a self-amplifying RNA vaccine against COVID-19: COVAC1, a phase I, dose-ranging trial. *EClinicalMedicine* 2022;44:101262. doi: 10.1016/j.eclinm.2021.101262.

89. Monin L, Laing AG, Muñoz-Ruiz M, et al. Safety and immunogenicity of one versus two doses of the COVID-19 vaccine BNT162b2 for patients with cancer: Interim analysis of a prospective observational study. *Lancet Oncol* 2021;22:765–778. doi: 10.1016/S1470-2045(21)00213-8.

90. Thomas SJ, Perez JL, Lockhart SP, et al. Efficacy and safety of the BNT162b2 mRNA COVID-19 vaccine in participants with a history of cancer: Subgroup analysis of a global phase 3 randomized clinical trial. *Vaccine* 2022;40:1483–1492. doi: 10.1016/j.vaccine.2021.12.046.

91. Hwang JK, Zhang T, Wang AZ, et al. COVID-19 vaccines for patients with cancer: Benefits likely outweigh risks. *J Hematol Oncol* 2021;14:38. doi: 10.1186/s13045-021-01046-w.

92. Fendler A, Shepherd STC, Au L, et al. Adaptive immunity and neutralizing antibodies against SARS-CoV-2 variants of concern following vaccination in patients with cancer: The CAPTURE study. *Nat Cancer* 2021;2:1321–1337. doi: 10.1038/s43018-021-00274-w.

93. Oosting SF, van der Veldt AAM, Geurtsvan Kessel CH, et al. mRNA-1273 COVID-19 vaccination in patients receiving chemotherapy, immunotherapy, or chemoimmunotherapy for solid tumours: A prospective, multicentre, non-inferiority trial. *Lancet Oncol* 2021;22:1681–1691. doi: 10.1016/S1470-2045(21)00574-X.

94. Cavanna L, Citterio C, Biasini C, et al. COVID-19 vaccines in adult cancer patients with solid tumours undergoing active treatment: Seropositivity and safety. A prospective observational study in Italy. *Eur J Cancer* 2021;157:441–449. doi: 10.1016/j.ejca.2021.08.035.

95. Peeters M, Verbruggen L, Teuwen L, et al. Reduced humoral immune response after BNT162b2 coronavirus disease 2019 messenger RNA vaccination in cancer patients under antineoplastic treatment. *ESMO Open* 2021;6:100274. doi: 10.1016/j.esmoop.2021.100274.

96. Shroff RT, Chalasani P, Wei R, et al. Immune responses to two and three doses of the BNT162b2 mRNA vaccine in adults with solid tumors. *Nat Med* 2021;27:2002–2011. doi: 10.1038/s41591-021-01542-z.

97. McKenzie DR, Muñoz-Ruiz M, Monin L, et al. Humoral and cellular immunity to delayed second dose of SARS-CoV-2 BNT162b2 mRNA vaccination in patients with cancer. *Cancer Cell* 2021;39:1445–1447. doi: 10.1016/j.ccell.2021.10.003.

98. Linardou H, Spanakis N, Koliou GA, et al. Responses to SARS-CoV-2 vaccination in patients with cancer (ReCOVer study): A prospective cohort study of the Hellenic cooperative oncology group. *Cancers* 2021;13:4621. doi: 10.3390/cancers13184621.

99. Shmueli ES, Itay A, Margalit O, et al. Efficacy and safety of BNT162b2 vaccination in patients with solid cancer receiving anticancer therapy – a single centre prospective study. *Eur J Cancer* 2021;157:124–131. doi: 10.1016/j.ejca.2021.08.007.

100. Agbarya A, Sarel I, Ziv-Baran T, et al. Efficacy of the mRNA-based BNT162b2 COVID-19 vaccine in patients with solid malignancies treated with anti-neoplastic drugs. *Cancers* 2021;13(16):4191. doi: 10.3390/cancers13164191.

101. Ligumsky H, Safadi E, Etan T, et al (2022) Immunogenicity and safety of the BNT162b2 mRNA COVID-19 vaccine among actively treated cancer patients. *J Natl Cancer Inst* 114:203–209. doi: 10.1093/jnci/djab174.

102. Barrière J, Chamorey E, Adjtoutah Z, et al. Impaired immunogenicity of BNT162b2 anti-SARS-CoV-2 vaccine in patients treated for solid tumors. *Ann Oncol* 2021;32:1053–1055. doi: 10.1016/j.annonc.2021.04.019.

103. Becerril-Gaitan A, Vaca-Cartagena BF, Ferrigno AS, et al. Immunogenicity and risk of severe acute respiratory syndrome coronavirus 2 (SARS-CoV-2) infection after coronavirus disease 2019 (COVID-19) vaccination in patients with cancer: A systematic review and meta-analysis. *Eur J Cancer* 2022;160:243–260. doi: 10.1016/j.ejca.2021.10.014.

104. Mair MJ, Berger JM, Berghoff AS, et al. Humoral immune response in hematooncological patients and health care workers who received SARS-CoV-2 vaccinations. *JAMA Oncol* 2022;8:106–113. doi: 10.1001/jamaoncol.2021.5437.

105. Embi PJ, Levy ME, Naleway AL, et al. Effectiveness of 2-dose vaccination with mRNA COVID-19 vaccines against COVID-19-associated hospitalizations among immunocompromised adults – Nine States, January–September 2021. *MMWR Morb Mortal Wkly Rep* 2021;70:1553–1559. doi: 10.15585/mmwr.mm7044e3.

106. Wu JT, La J, Branch-Elliman W, et al. Association of COVID-19 vaccination with SARS-CoV-2 infection in patients with cancer: A US nationwide veterans affairs study. *JAMA Oncol* 2022; 8:281–286. doi: 10.1001/jamaoncol.2021.5771.

107. Hippisley-Cox J, Coupland CA, Mehta N, et al. Risk prediction of COVID-19 related death and hospital admission in adults after COVID-19 vaccination: National prospective cohort study. *BMJ* 2021;374:n2244. doi: 10.1136/bmj.n2244. Erratum in: BMJ 2021 Sep 20;374:n2300.

108. Zeng C, Evans JP, Chakravarthy K, et al. COVID-19 mRNA booster vaccines elicit strong protection against SARS-CoV-2 Omicron variant in patients with cancer. *Cancer Cell* 2021;40:117–119. doi: 10.1016/j.ccell.2021.12.014.

109. Valanparambil R, Carlisle J, Linderman S, et al. Antibody response to SARS-CoV-2 mRNA vaccine in lung cancer patients: Reactivity to vaccine antigen and variants of concern. medRxiv [Preprint] doi: 10.1101/2022.01.03.22268599. Update in: Antibody response to COVID-19 mRNA vaccine in patients with lung cancer after primary immunization and booster: Reactivity to the SARS-CoV-2 WT virus and omicron variant. *J Clin Oncol* 2022;40(33):3808–3816. doi: 10.1200/JCO.21.02986.

110. Fendler A, Shepherd STC, Au L, et al. CAPTURE consortium. Omicron neutralising antibodies after third COVID-19 vaccine dose in patients with cancer. *Lancet* 2022;399:905–907. doi: 10.1016/S0140-6736(22)00147-7.

111. Thakkar A, Gonzalez-Lugo JD, Goradia N, et al. Seroconversion rates following COVID-19 vaccination among patients with cancer. *Cancer Cell* 2021;39:1081–1090.e2. doi: 10.1016/j.ccell.2021.06.002.

112. Massarweh A, Eliakim-Raz N, Stemmer A, et al. Evaluation of seropositivity following BNT162b2 messenger RNA vaccination for SARS-CoV-2 in patients undergoing treatment for cancer. *JAMA Oncol* 2021;7:1133–1140. doi: 10.1001/jamaoncol.2021.2155.

113. Ehmsen S, Asmussen A, Jeppesen SS, et al. Antibody and T cell immune responses following mRNA COVID-19 vaccination in patients with cancer. *Cancer Cell* 2021;39:1034–1036. doi: 10.1016/j.ccell.2021.07.016.

114. Mairhofer M, Kausche L, Kaltenbrunner S, et al. Humoral and cellular immune responses in SARS-CoV-2 mRNA-vaccinated patients with cancer. *Cancer Cell* 2021;39:1171–1172. doi: 10.1016/j.ccell.2021.08.001.

115. Karacin C, Eren T, Zeynelgil E, et al (2021) Immunogenicity and safety of the CoronaVac vaccine in patients with cancer receiving active systemic therapy. *Future Oncol* 17:4447–4456. doi: 10.2217/fon-2021-0597.

116. Ariamanesh M, Porouhan P, PeyroShabany B, et al. Immunogenicity and Safety of the Inactivated SARS-CoV-2 Vaccine (BBIBP-CorV) in Patients with Malignancy. *Cancer Invest* 2022;40:26–34. doi: 10.1080/07357907.2021.1992420.

117. Addeo A, Shah PK, Bordry N, et al. Immunogenicity of SARS-CoV-2 messenger RNA vaccines in patients with cancer. *Cancer Cell* 2021;39:1091–1098.e2. doi: 10.1016/j.ccell.2021.06.009.

118. Matkowska-Kocjan A, Owoc-Lempach J, Chruszcz J, et al. The COVID-19 mRNA BNT163b2 vaccine was well tolerated and highly immunogenic in young adults in long follow-up after haematopoietic stem cell transplantation. *Vaccines* 2021;9:1209. doi: 10.3390/vaccines9101209.

119. Malard F, Gaugler B, Gozlan J, et al. Weak immunogenicity of SARS-CoV-2 vaccine in patients with hematologic malignancies. *Blood Cancer J* 2021;11:142. doi: 10.1038/s41408-021-00534-z.

120. Liebers N, Speer C, Benning L, et al. Humoral and cellular responses after COVID-19 vaccination in anti-CD20-treated lymphoma patients. *Blood* 2022;139:142–147. doi: 10.1182/blood.2021013445.

121. Aleman A, Upadhyaya B, Tuballes K, et al. Variable cellular responses to SARS-CoV-2 in fully vaccinated patients with multiple myeloma. *Cancer Cell* 2021;39:1442–1444. doi: 10.1016/j.ccell.2021.09.015.

122. Marasco V, Carniti C, Guidetti A, et al. T-cell immune response after mRNA SARS-CoV-2 vaccines is frequently detected also in the absence of seroconversion in patients with lymphoid malignancies. *Br J Haematol* 2022;196:548–558. doi: 10.1111/bjh.17877.

123. Bange EM, Han NA, Wileyto P, et al. CD8+T cells contribute to survival in patients with COVID-19 and hematologic cancer. *Nat Med* 2021;27:1280–1289. doi: 10.1038/s41591-021-01386-7.

124. Fendler A, Au L, Shepherd STC, et al. Functional antibody and T cell immunity following SARS-CoV-2 infection, including by variants of concern, in patients with cancer: The CAPTURE study. *Nat Cancer* 2021;2:1321–1337. doi: 10.1038/s43018-021-00275-9.

125. Fendler A, de Vries EGE, Geurtsvan Kessel CH, et al. COVID-19 vaccines in patients with cancer: Immunogenicity, efficacy and safety. *Nat Rev Clin Oncol* 2022;19:385–401. doi: 10.1038/s41571-022-00610-8.

11

Air Pollution and COVID-19: A Synergistic Effect Accelerating Male Infertility and Cancer

Luigi Montano, Marina Piscopo, Carlo Brogna, and Maria Luisia Chiusano

Air Pollution and Diseases

Air pollution is among the major concerns in both industrialised and underdeveloped world regions [1]. Several epidemiological studies consider air pollution a major risk factor for non-communicable diseases, premature deaths, and reproduction dysfunctions, as reviewed by Manisalidis et al. [2].

The European Environmental Agency [3] reports that the percentage of the European population exposed to concentrations of main atmospheric pollutants above the World Health Organization (WHO) guidelines in 2017 at 77.2% in case of particulate matter (PM) with a diameter of less than 2.5 micron (PM2.5) (fine dust), 44.4% for PM10 (fine dust, thin with a diameter between 10 and 2.5 micron), 95.9% for ozone (O3), and 6.5% for nitrogen dioxide (NO2). Such values were in relative improvement compared to 2006, which recorded 97.4% of the population exposed to PM2.5, 85.6% to PM10, 99% to O3, and 18.2% to NO2.

The European Environment Agency also reports [3] the 76,200 early deaths from air pollution in Italy. Of these, 58,600 were attributed to airborne fine particulate matter, 3,000 to O3, and 14,600 to NO2. The figures are by far the highest in Europe, even higher (in absolute value) than in Germany, a nation with nearly 25 million more habitants than Italy.

The American Lung Association [4] indicated the following effects resulting from exposure to air pollutants:

- respiratory and cardiovascular problems (including strokes);
- increased mortality in infants and children;
- increase in the number of heart attacks
- inflammation of lung tissue in young, healthy adults;
- increased visits to the emergency room for patients with acute respiratory disorders;
- increased hospitalisation for asthma in children;
- increased severity of asthma attacks in children; and
- cerebrovascular diseases.

DOI: 10.1201/9781003362562-12

In addition, impact on male fertility and cancer must be considered because of their impact on quality of life, health management, and progeny.

Already in 1995, Seaton et al [5] proposed that ultra-fine acid particles, characteristic of atmospheric pollution, would cause alveolar inflammation, changes in blood coagulability, and release of mediators capable of causing acute respiratory syndromes in sensitive individuals. In addition, the work points out that blood coagulability increases the susceptibility of individuals to cardiovascular disease.

Frampton et al [6] observed that the inhalation of ultrafine atmospheric particulate is responsible for systemic inflammation and vasoconstriction, which can lead to the overexpression of pro-inflammatory cytokines and a series of events that cause thrombosis. Worthy to note, systemic inflammation and the induction of blood clotting, resulting in thrombotic and thromboembolic effects, are the same pathological findings highlighted by the autopsies of COVID-19 patients [7].

Ross [8] reports that long exposures to fine particles cause blood clotting, hypertension, and vascular reactivity, while Russell and Brunekreef [9] (2009) highlighted that the effects on the lung are associated with cell damage and inflammation. Growing evidence points out that reactive oxygen species (ROS), both present in fine particles and produced by stimulated cells, play an important role in these processes.

Air pollution can also increase the incidence and risk of mortality from cerebrovascular diseases [10]. The authors found a statistically significant correlation between stroke mortality and the level of air pollution in the city of Como, in relationship with the concentration of PM10 and NO2 in the months of December, January, and February, the typical period of the flu epidemic. Interestingly, Como was one of the Italian cities more affected by COVID-19 in 2020, with a mortality increase of 23.4% (ISTAT, 2021).

The mechanisms of cardiovascular disease, lung oxidative stress, and particulate matter–related inflammation have been described in a recent review in rodent models [11]. This work shows that chronic exposure to PM2.5 not only causes inflammation in the alveolar district, but by crossing the alveolar barrier, reaches the blood and thus peripheral tissues, leading to oxidative stress either directly or through excessive production of ROS. This leads to inflammasome activation, in particular NLRP3, which affects cytokine maturation and secretion, like interleukins IL-1 beta and IL-18, which are all implicated in inflammatory systemic syndromes and in conditions that promote the virulence of pathogens, such as vascular discharge and coagulopathies [12]. Therefore, it is conceivable that the inflammatory mediators generated in the lungs as a result of air pollutants could exert a systemic effect and also have the potential to promote silent systemic inflammation. Indeed, evidence of systemic oxidative stress has been observed following exposure to atmospheric particulates [13].

Air Pollution, Male Fertility and Transgenerational Effects

The prevalence of male infertility has increased significantly (from 7 to 8% in the 1960s to 20–30% today), and several studies have revealed that sperm concentration has dropped in many industrialised countries over the past few decades. Carlsen examined the semen analyses of donor samples from 1934 to 1990 in a meta-analysis of 61 European studies conducted in 1992, and he noted a progressive deterioration of the semen's qualitative and quantitative characteristics (from 113 Mil/mL in 1940 to

66 Mil/mL in 1990 and a 19% decline in ejaculate volume) [14]. Men's sperm concentration (SC) and total sperm count (TSC), specifically in North America, Europe, and Australia, fell considerably between 1973 and 2011, according to a systematic review and meta-regression model [15]. Recently a new meta-analysis by Levine et al reported how sperm count is declining at an accelerated pace globally [16].

Male reproductive health is currently significantly impacted by a number of environmental factors, including air pollution and endocrine-disrupting substances, which can alter the normal hormonal balance [17–19], and/or induce oxidative stress and/or genetic and epigenetic changes [20].

Numerous epidemiological research indicates that the hormonal unbalancing has a deleterious impact on semen parameters [20, 21]. Through excessive ROS–mediated autophagy that destroys tight junctions, adherens junctions, and gap junctions, a recent experimental study on rats shows that PM2.5 alters the integrity of the blood–testis barrier [22]. It has been noted that continuous exposure to NO2 and SO2 is negatively associated with sperm count, motility, and even testicular volume in infertile people, revealing the detrimental effects of specific pollutants on spermatogenesis. Additionally, it has been reported that lower levels of SO2 enhance spermatogenesis [23]. A Chinese pre-proof study recently found that exposure to particulate matter with a diameter equal to or fewer than 10 microns (PM10) during spermatidogenesis (from 6 to 12 weeks) is associated with reduced sperm concentration and total and progressive motility of spermatozoa, using linear multivariate distributed lag models to identify windows of exposure to air pollution susceptibility during the spermatogenic cycle [24]. While exposure to O3 during the spermiogenesis period (11 to 12 weeks) was associated with low sperm count, exposure to SO2 during the spermatocytogenesis period (0 to 5 weeks) had a negative correlation with sperm concentration and total spermatozoa motility. In animal models, chronic exposure to PM2.5 has been shown to suppress the hypothalamus-pituitary-gonad axis (HPG) and result in a significant decrease in follicle-stimulating hormone (FSH), low circulating testosterone, and consequently reduced sperm concentration [25, 26]. All of these findings supported the hypothesis that air pollution affects all phases of the spermatogenetic cycle through many routes [27], supporting the epidemiological evidence that it may affect one or more seminal parameters [28].

Numerous studies have shown also that exposure to air pollutants can cause genetic damage to male germ cells [29], and epidemiological studies have shown that the quality of human sperm may reflect men's health status [30–33]. The first systematic study on the effect of air pollution on human health, carried out in the Czech Republic as part of the "Teplice" research programme, discovered higher DNA fragmentation and sperm aneuploidy rates. High levels of polycyclic aromatic hydrocarbons (PAHs) and PM10 in the air, as well as the frequent detection of air pollutants in semen, were linked to both effects [34]. The authors postulated that DNA adducts made by PAHs might be present in the semen of those exposed to high levels of pollution, leading to increased sperm DNA fragmentation [35]. After periods of exposure to both low and high intermittent air pollution, Rubes and colleagues validated the role of air pollutants in sperm DNA damage in young boys, still in Teplice [36]. Recent molecular analyses from co-authors of this chapter revealed that sperm nuclear basic proteins from samples of males living in polluted locations had a novel and unexpected behaviour, being engaged in oxidative DNA damage [37]. Animal studies have also demonstrated epigenetic effects on male gametes of particulate matter, particularly those associated with DNA methylation [38]. Heavy metals can build up in human semen, and studies have linked them to sperm quality characteristics such as motility, morphology, DNA strand integrity, telomere length, and DNA methylation [39–42]. The common factor via which air pollutants can cause damages at the biomolecular level, including DNA, proteins, and lipids, leading to chronic low-grade inflammation, may be oxidative stress due to an excess of reactive oxygen species (ROS), imbalanced by the existence of reductive activity [21, 43]. Due to the abundance of polyunsaturated fatty acids in their plasma membrane, which are known to be ROS targets, and the low intracytoplasmic presence of antioxidant enzymes resulting from the small cytoplasmic volume, spermatozoa are extremely sensitive to the pro-oxidant action of contaminants [41].

ACE2, the angiotensin-converting enzyme 2, the membrane protein able to interact with SARS-CoV-2 permitting the viral entry into the human cells [44], is also present in the male reproductive system. It is also known to control the inflammatory response in lungs under exposure to PM2.5 [45]. Therefore, it should be of interest to investigate the effects of particulate matter on testes or changes in the sperm physiology in relationship to ACE2 concentration and in knockout experiments.

Sensitivity to a number of pollutants has been demonstrated to grow from generation to generation in mice [46], and preliminary findings suggest transgenerational effects of pollutants due to molecular changes at sperm level in humans from polluted areas [47]. Of special interest is the increased susceptibility to non-communicable diseases (NCDs) and the marked decrease in defense systems in the body. Overall, this appears to provide a revised explanation for the worldwide disease burden, and this could also be understood not merely by a chronic-degenerative approach, but also as resulting from involvement of contagious pathogens (dengue, yellow fever, and so on) [46, 48–50]. As a matter of fact, experimental data have demonstrated, indeed, that dioxins and other contaminants have the potential to affect the host's immune response, which can be transmitted to successive generations, decreasing the ability of the host to protect against viral pathogens [46, 48–50].

Air Pollution And Cancer

While it has been sufficiently demonstrated that air pollution has direct effects on the respiratory system and that it increases the risk of lung cancer even in non-smokers [51–54], there are few studies that associate air pollution with increased mortality for different types of cancer. A study carried out in the urban and suburban areas of Hong Kong examined 66,820 people aged 65 and monitored the mortality outcomes between 1998 and 2011, simultaneously considering the annual concentrations of PM on the basis of their residence, concluding that long-term exposure to PM2.5 was associated with several types of cancer [55].

A recent systematic review and meta-analysis of epidemiological studies published from 1980 to 2021, evaluating the association of PM2.5 and PM10 with gastrointestinal cancer incidence or mortality, showed a strong association between particulate matter levels and gastrointestinal cancers, particularly with liver and colorectal cancers [56].

The most plausible biological mechanisms of PM damage in inducing the carcinogenic process appear to be: (i) oxidative stress with subsequent damage to DNA, proteins, and lipids; (ii) inflammation effect directly or indirectly induced by PM, leading to the production of chemokine and cytokines; and (iii) epigenetic modifications such as DNA methylation, histone modifications, and noncoding RNA expression [55, 57].

SARS-CoV-2 Mediated Damages

Like SARS-CoV, SARS-CoV-2 uses the angiotensin-converting enzyme 2 (ACE2) as its receptor to enter cells [44]. This causes mild, moderate, moderately severe, to extremely critical forms of COVID-19. Even more, the asymptomatic forms of the disease can also determine the viral transmission. The receptor ACE2 has a key role in the renin-angiotensin-aldosterone-system (RAAS), the complex system that regulates blood pressure, converting the hormone angiotensin II (ANGII) into angiotensin 1–7 (ANG [1–7]) [58, 59].

COVID-19 symptoms have been mainly linked to effects on ACE2 enzyme activity [60]. In COVID-19 patients, inactivation of the ACE2 complex causes abnormal sensory and neurological perception, thrombosis in both infected and uninfected tissues, and, most critically, necrosis in pulmonary, endothelial, and cardiac cells. In addition, blood pressure regulation can be affected. The severe pulmonary and the systemic clinical pictures point to a hyperinflammatory syndrome known as hemophagocytic lymphohistiocytosis, with a cytokine storm characterised by elevated levels of IL-2, IL-7, granulocyte-inducing factors (granulocyte colony-stimulating factor), interferon, inducible protein 10, monocyte chemoattractant protein 1, macrophage inflammatory protein 1, and TNF-alpha (tumor necrosis factor-alpha) [60, 139]. The mechanisms of damage at pulmonary level are similar to those caused by the 2009 influenza A (H1N1) and by the avian (H5M1) viruses, which initiate a process of immune dysregulation, with overproduction of cytokines [60], generally provoking ARDS (acute respiratory distress syndrome).

The Italian Society of Vascular Diagnostics and the Italian Society of Vascular Medicine [61] included, among the pathologies attributed to the SARS-Cov-2 infection, the inflammation as a cause of coagulopathy and of the synergy between coagulopathy and viral infection. The authors recall how the correlation between inflammation and coagulation has been widely demonstrated, in the sense that an inflammatory process can cause an alteration of coagulation through the activation of inflammatory cytokines, among other events. Burstein [62] pointed out the possible negative role of cytokines on the hemostatic system and on thrombogenesis, and, two years later, Esmon et al [63] recalled how the mechanism linking inflammation and coagulation was established beyond any reasonable doubt. In addition, Esmon [64] described the stages of the interaction between inflammation and coagulation, the initiation of coagulation, the decrease in the activity of natural anticoagulant mechanisms, and damage to the fibrinolytic system, underlining that inflammatory cytokines are the main mediators involved in the activation of coagulation. This highlights the vicious circle between increased inflammation and increased blood clotting, which in turn increases inflammation because of the inability of natural anticoagulant mechanisms to control the process. This suggests that anticoagulants may represent an effective treatment in the case of acute inflammatory syndromes. Considering the synergy between coagulopathy and viral infection, it should be recalled that this syndrome has been known at least since 1967, when McKay and Margaretten [65] indicated the disseminated intravascular coagulation due to viral infections, suggesting an appropriate anticoagulant therapy to decrease morbidity and mortality.

Recent reports of viral infection of endothelial cells also resulted in endotheliitis, a severe inflammatory reaction, and systemic impairment of microcirculatory function. Multiple organ dysfunction is caused by these pathogenetic processes [66, 67]. Indeed, it was reported that also liver, lungs, brain, spleen, pancreas, and jejunum all showed elevated amounts of TNF-alpha, interleukin-6, and interleukin-8 [68]. An immune-mediated reaction determines also the possible damage at central nervous system (CNS) level [69]. For instance, IL-6 production in the CNS has been linked to convulsions [70], while TNF-alpha is known to enhance blood-brain barrier permeability and trigger cell death [71].

These findings demonstrate that extra-respiratory tissues actively participate in the proinflammatory cytokine response during severe infections, which may aggravate the patient's clinical conditions with possible fatal outcomes.

It has been demonstrated that many viruses, SARS-CoV-2 in particular, can quickly cause an autoimmune dysregulation by triggering a considerable cytokine production in genetically predisposed individuals, primarily TNF-alpha, IL-6 and IL-1, IL-17, and IL-18, [72]. This process might be even more critical if exposure to environmental impacts affects the regulatory systems that drive cytokine synthesis and release, causing dysregulation and overproduction with an excess of innate and adaptive response mechanisms [73, 74]. Additionally, as in specific populations or ethnic groups, cytokine release and/or the presence of particular IL-6 polymorphisms may make people more vulnerable to viral issues [75]. It is interesting to note that secondary hemophagocytic lymphohistiocytosis (sHLH) and an increase in interferon (IFN), IL-1, and IL-6 signatures are brought on by pulmonary involvement in individuals with juvenile systemic idiopathic arthritis (SJIA) [76, 77]. Noteworthy is the claim by Mehta et al that COVID-19 severity is linked to a cytokine storm condition resembling sHLH [78]. According to a previous theory, environmental variables may also cause or worsen an abnormal innate and acquired immune response with large cytokine production in genetically vulnerable people with sHLH [79].

Pollution and SARS-CoV-2

Currently, many studies suggest that air pollution may play a significant role in determining the rate of COVID-19 outbreak spread and mortality [97], particularly in cities with high levels of air pollutants where other unfavourable conditions like higher temperatures and humidity, greater population density [80], and commercial exchanges [81] (both of the latter which account for human-to-human transmission mechanisms) play a significant role in the outbreak. The theory holds that certain environmental factors, especially indoors and air pollutants, may encourage the persistence of viruses in the atmosphere. This observation has been made for both the coronavirus SARS-CoV, spread during the 2003 infection [82], and SARS-CoV-2 [80], and it has been claimed that it may encourage both indirect and direct (person-to-individual) dissemination. Although this has not yet been fully explored, putatively also for economical interests, several articles have hypothesised that the interaction of PMs with the virus may provide a possible higher risk of virus propagation [83–85]. In China, during the SARS outbreak in 2003, a relationship between air pollution indexes and SARS case mortalities was already noted, with the death rate being twice as high in the most polluted areas towards the least polluted ones [86]. After correcting for relative humidity and temperature readings, Wuhan, China, faced a greater CFR (case fatality rate) for COVID-19 with rising time-scaled air particulate matter concentrations (PM10 and PM2.5) [87]. While pointing out that factors like population size, elderly population, extreme poverty, and income level can affect the spread of COVID-19, a very recent study of 615 cities on six continents also revealed that PM2.5, NO2, and O3 under specific meteorological conditions such as dew, wind gust, pressure, and wind speed increase the spread of COVID-19, promoting its detrimental health effects and higher mortality rates [88]. In support of these evidences, the fatality rates for SARS-CoV-2 transmission are notably higher in industrial areas with the worst pollution levels [89–92]. In Europe, a study of 66 administrative regions in Spain, Italy, France, and Germany using geographical analysis revealed a 78% CFR (3487 on 4443 fatality cases). The highest CFR for COVID-19 among western nations was in central Spain and five regions of the Po Valley, in northern Italy, both of which have incredibly high levels of particulate matter such as PM10, PM2.5, and nitric dioxide (NO2) [93–95]. A frequent common characteristic of COVID-19 and air pollution is increased mortality from cardiovascular and pulmonary disorders. Pozzer and coworkers [96] calculated the anthropogenic proportion based on satellite data to characterise global fine particle exposure and estimated the COVID-19 mortality that may be attributed to long-term exposure to fine particulate air pollution. According to their research, anthropogenic air pollution was responsible for 15% of COVID-19-related deaths worldwide, ~27% in East Asia, ~19% in Europe, and ~17% in North America. Most fascinatingly, mortality from COVID-19 attributed to all anthropogenic pollutants was found to be 3% in Australia, where air quality standards do not permit yearly PM2.5 values above 8 mg/m^3. Indeed, the weighted population exposure to PM2.5 and the geographical areas with a high mortality fraction appear correlated. Noticeably, the influence of climatic factors such as temperature, precipitation, and humidity on the spread of viruses, particularly for respiratory syncytial virus (RSV) bronchiolitis, has been matter of attention to prevent outbreaks in specific areas [97]. Interestingly, ACE2 knockout animals had higher levels of resting respiratory rate (RRR), IL-6, TGF-1, TNF-, and MMP9 than wild-type animals when exposed to inhalation of PM2.5, indicating that ACE2 may play a protective role against the PM2.5–induced inflammatory process [45]. ACE2 expression levels also increased in PM2.5–exposed wild-type animals. Therefore, the sequestration of ACE2, due to SARS-CoV-2 infection, may contribute additional mechanisms that enhance the inflammatory effects associated with the viral infection [58].

Male Fertility, Air Pollution, and COVID-19

Despite the fact that environmental pollution is everywhere, there are some regions of the world where higher levels of environmental stress are associated with higher rates of infertility and chronic degenerative disorders. Additionally, this relationship can be discovered within countries or even within the same county/region [98, 99].

Since the 1950s, in France, there has been a rise in the general population's exposure to chemicals [100]. All of the main endocrine-disrupting chemicals (EDCs) have been found in the biological matrices of French people, and some of them (non-dioxin-like PCBs, pesticides, and triclosan) were found in higher amounts than in individuals from other countries [101]. Similar shreds of evidence are available from the "Land of Fires," in the Campania Region, Italy, where the rising prevalence of abnormalities of the male reproductive system has drawn attention to the potential environmental risk factors [39]. These findings support the recent assertion made in a global report that endocrine disruptors play a significant role in decreased semen quality [102]. Therefore, changes in the environmental exposure of males living in highly polluted areas and a potential transgenerational effect may be to blame for the global decline in sperm concentration and shape, at least in part [102].

For human and marine species living in high environmental impact areas this is a health risk [103–106], as spermatozoa are the first to be harmed by environmental insults and can be thought of as early and sensitive markers of environmental exposures. In addition, spermatozoa may be particularly vulnerable to the effects of SARS-CoV-2 since human semen is an early and sensitive health marker [107] which could further raise the likelihood of infertility in the affected male population. Reproductive biomarkers, particularly seminal biomarkers, could thus serve as good biological indicators for the assessment of environmental harm to human health, including male fertility, in addition to the assessment of virulence and severity of viral effect [107, 108].

These aspects are important, especially in subjects at the age of their peak reproductive activity, around 30 years, when the expression levels of ACE2 receptors are higher than in subjects aged 20 or 60 []. Nevertheless, there is still lack of clinical data on the short- and long-term effects of the current virus on the male reproductive system, and the role of the renin-angiotensin system also in testes and epididymis and on spermatogenesis [109].

A "double-hit theory" was put forth by several authors in an effort to theorise how environmental contamination can worsen COVID-19 symptoms [110]. Chronic PM2.5 exposure increases alveolar ACE2 receptor over-expression, which results in predisposition to SARS-CoV-2 infection, inflammation, and possible ACE2 receptor depletion. In turn, this may increase local viral load in pollutant-exposed patients. High atmospheric NO2 concentrations may provide a second blow, resulting in a severe COVID-19 infection in ACE-2-depleted lungs and a subsequent deterioration of the prognosis [111]. Theoretically, the effects of COVID-19 on male fertility could be greater in polluted areas, where higher pollutant levels may increase the severity of SARS-CoV-2 infection [112] and explain the negative effects on male fertility caused by deleterious synergic effects due to the simultaneous presence of air pollution and the virus. This evidence could also be applied to the male reproductive system. High local physiological levels of the ACE2 enzyme in the testis, which have been found to increase in the testicles of infertile men [113], may play a protective role by acting in two different ways: (i) by lowering AngII(1–8) levels and reducing its signaling through the AT1 receptor; and (ii) by generating Ang(1–7), which activates the Mas-receptor–dependent pathway and reduces the deleterious effects of high levels of PM2.5 in polluted environments. Nevertheless, it may have negative synergistic effects with the SARS-CoV-2 infection. In addition to the excessive ROS–mediated autophagy already described [25], PM2.5 may raise the already high levels of ACE2, which may favor the viral entry into the cell, accompanied by the enzyme inactivation.

This results in cell death, and in a decrease in the production of Ang(1–9), which would lead to an accumulation of AngI(1–10); another would be an accumulation of AngII(1–8); a severe overactivation of the ACE/AngI-AngII/AT1R pathway with all the associated effects; and a fourth would be a decrease in the ACE2/Ang-(1–7)/MasR pathway. When combined, these processes would result in a significant inflammatory response and undermine the physiological effects of MasR signaling on spermatogenesis, the chance of apoptosis, inflammatory processes, an excessive creation of reactive oxygen species (ROS), and immunoregulatory system activation [114, 115].

However, more investigation is required to conclusively show the presence of the virus in the male reproductive system and, in case, its persistence after the acute infection phase.

There may be other factors that affect fertility. Pollutants and RNA viruses both have intracellular targets that are largely mitochondria, which are found in great abundance in spermatozoa. Mitochondrial DNA is extremely sensitive to the effects of pollutants, and in its very early stages of intracellular invasion, SARS-CoV-2 has been shown to interact with certain mitochondrial proteins, whose down-regulation appears to determine an energy dysfunction with changes in the oxide/reductive balance, i.e., the induction of excessive production of reactive oxygen species (ROS), an inflammatory process, an alteration of apoptosis, and immunoregulatory mechanisms [114, 115].

COVID-19 and Cancer

There are three aspects to be taken into account when considering the relationship between cancer and COVID-19, such as increased risk of infection and worsening of the disease. Cancer is considered one of the factors that can increase susceptibility to COVID-19 [116]. Vice versa, people suffering from cancer seem to exhibit exacerbated conditions and have higher mortality rates when exposed to SARS-Cov-2.

Earlier published reports indicated that patients who had comorbidities were at a greater mortality risk or were at higher incidence to develop more severe forms of COVID-19. Specifically, people of any age with certain medical conditions are at increased risk of severe illness from COVID-19. Among the diseases, chronic kidney disease, chronic obstructive pulmonary disease (COPD), obesity, serious heart conditions, anemia sickle cell disease, type 2 diabetes, and cancer are listed [117]. However, the patients suffering from cancer are usually more susceptible to infections and therefore to SARS-CoV-2. In particular, when compared to the overall population, cancer patients have about three times the vulnerability to death from COVID-19 as their immune systems may be weakened by cancer and its treatments [118]. This trial was conducted in 105 cancer patients and 536 age-matched non-cancer patients with COVID-19. Cancer patients have a high relative mortality rate, high rate of intensive care unit admission, high probability of using invasive mechanical ventilation, and a higher risk to develop serious symptoms than non-cancer patients, as a consequence of COVID-19. In addition, a study of 1,524 cancer patients who were screened at Zhongnan Hospital of Wuhan University have a higher risk of SARS-CoV infection compared with the community [117]. People affected by cancer can have an increased risk of infection to COVID-19, which can be linked to a weakened immune system [119]. Tumours, including lymphoma and leukemia, can lead to thrombocytopenia, caused by imbalance of thrombopoiesis, and loss of platelet function and integrity.

Thus, the platelet's role in eradicating viruses by direct and indirect mechanisms involving presentation of the pathogen to the innate and adaptive immune systems is compromised [120]. However, there must be also considered that, although the majority of evidence supports a significantly greater risk of severe COVID-19 in patients with active cancer as adults [121–123], data are contradictory [124–126] and the outcomes are improved through better COVID-19 therapy and an earlier diagnosis [127]. The risk probably differs based on the type and stage of the tumor and the treatment received. In detail, the following features have been linked to higher risk.

- Haematologic diseases or lung cancer [127–139]. An aspect to be noted is the hypercoagulation status, present in both cancer patients [140] and COVID-19 patients, highlighted by the increase of D-dimer and C-reaction protein (PCR) [141]. Some authors have elucidated the compression of the arachidonic pathway with a hyper level of prostaglandins (PGs) [142]. The impairment of the arachidonic acid pathway is also affected by a marked presence of phospholipase A2 in sufferers [143]. Some studies have shown that these effects may be related to gut microbiome disruption [144]. On the other hand, gut dysbiosis is correlated with increased cancers in particular groups, such as breast cancer [145] or colorectal cancer [146].

Risk factors that were in association with worsening overall survival in the patients having haematologic neoplasms and COVID-19 included older age, a progressive illness status, a diagnosis of acute myeloid leukemia, non-Hodgkin's indolent lymphoma, and aggressive non-Hodgkin's lymphoma or plasma cell neoplasms, and serious or more critical COVID-19. In addition, patients were at highest risk of death independent of whether they had a recent illness or were receiving specific therapy or both. The rate of death in patients who had haematological neoplasms and COVID-19 was elevated as compared with the overall population who had COVID-19 and patients that had haematological malignancies but did not have COVID-19 [147]. Similar results were reported by other authors, in which COVID-19 patients affected by haematologic neoplasms possessed a mortality rate significantly higher than that for patients without cancer. The associated risk factors of mortality included age (>70 years) and concentration of C-reactive protein (>10 mg/dl). Treatment with active chemotherapy and the viral load upon diagnosis did not predict worse outcomes in these patients [148, 149].

- Advanced and/or progressive cancer [119, 123, 129, 150–155]. Chemotherapy-active treatments, especially myelosuppressive regimens are also discussed, even though there are conflicting data [153, 154, 156, 157]. By contrast, the recent immuno-therapy seems not to worsen the outcomes of COVID-19 [158–160], albeit again the data are conflicting [161]. Advanced age [125, 126, 153, 154, 162, 163] and concurrent conditions [161, 164–174] that are associated with severe COVID-19 in an independent manner additionally contribute to the risk in patients with cancer. Nevertheless, at least one extensive meta-analysis was reported to propose that younger cancer patients are at higher risk of worsening COVID-19 outcomes than similarly aged controls with no cancer [138]. However, to date, researchers have found that among patients younger than 25 years of age who have cancer and COVID-19, risk factors of severe infection include lymphopenia, newly administered steroids, chimeric antigen receptor-modified T-cell therapy (CAR-T), and elevated viral load [175].

Some evidence supports the idea that being a previous cancer survivor is also a risk factor for severe COVID-19; however, the risks are lower than for active cancer [129, 168, 176], whereas some other studies have not found higher risks among survivors [153, 177].

On the other hand, patients suffering from cancer also experience associated health conditions, caused by their status, including heart disease, diabetes, dyslipidemia, hypertension, obesity, osteoporosis, osteopenia, and mental illnesses (major depressive disorder and generalised anxiety disorder) [178]. Among these, hypertension and hyperlipidemia were the two most common comorbidities at 70% and over 50% respectively [179], followed by some heart-related conditions. This overlaps the most frequent comorbidities in COVID-19. Thus, emerging research demonstrates a worse trend among COVID-19 cancer patients compared with non–COVID-19 cancer patients. Nevertheless, other evidence also suggests that the rates of SARS-CoV-2 infection and severe events in cancer patients are not higher compared with the general population. Thus, the investigations being conducted are necessary to better clarify the comorbidity of COVID-19 and cancer. Since the majority of reports associated with cancer patients having COVID-19 have involved cohort studies of a relatively small sample size, limited clinical information, and high heterogeneity of tumor stages and cancer types, as well as different treatments, current understanding is still limited. Thus, clinical outcomes and biological basis for cancer comorbidity and COVID-19 remain to be elucidated.

The potential for the recurrence of COVID-19 leads to an emerging sense of the need to explore new strategies to improve the management and care of patients that have cancer with COVID-19. Moreover, additional data showed the prevalence of cancer among COVID-19 patients with a variable range from 1% to 6% in Asian populations and up to 18% in Western countries [180]. In addition, some researches demonstrate that COVID-19 enhances complications and total risk of dying in cancer patients [119, 153, 181]. Nevertheless, such analyses were limited due to the sample size and the intrinsic bias of screened symptomatic patients. The evidence from China, albeit limited in sample size, indicated that the patients who had cancer worsened faster than those without cancer and had an increased risk of severe complications from COVID-19, including death [119, 153, 181]. More recent findings from the UK collaboration OPENSafely (~6,000 deaths due to COVID-19) [182] corroborates previous evidence showing a three-fold increased risk of death in patients with a diagnosis of hematologic malignancy up to 5 years preceding SARS-CoV infection. The increased risk of death seemed to be lower for other types of cancer than for hematologic malignancies, but it also was similarly significant (hazard 1.56), mainly for those diagnosed with cancer within 1 year of SARS-CoV-2 infection [182, 183]. Finally, in a prospective cohort study of a total of 1,035 cancer patients (mean age of 66 years) who had COVID-19, the most predominant malignancies were found to be breast and prostate cancer [153]. Thirteen percent of the patients were dead by four weeks after the diagnosis of COVID-19. Several prognostic factors were linked to the mortality related to COVID-19 in these oncologic patients. Age (deaths increased with age), gender (more males died or were hospitalised in the ICU compared with females), status as a smoker (more current or former smokers died), the number of comorbidities (a greater proportion of comorbidities were associated with more deaths), types of malignancy (more solid tumor patients died than those who had haematologic cancer), and tumor status. Nevertheless, race, ethnicity, obesity, types, or malignancy, or treatment of cancer factors, were not related to mortality [153, 184].

In this context, there is the question: Does air pollution cause cancer? Does COVID-19 cause cancer? Does the cancer-inflamed state worsen with COVID-19? In this regard, it should also be considered that air pollution is a major contributor to lung cancer [185]. Oncology patients are most vulnerable for COVID-19-related disease, and multiple associated risk factors are ascribed to the severity of the disease. Furthermore, it appears that cancer treatments do not associate with COVID-19 severity, which could benefit the well-being of oncology patients in this pandemic [186]. Moreover, long COVID-19 may predispose recovered patients to the development of cancer and accelerate its progression. This hypothesis has been based on the increasing evidence of the capacity of SARS-CoV-2 to modulate oncogenic pathways, induce chronic low-grade inflammation, and promote tissue damage. For this reason, extensive research is urgently required to clarify the impact of long COVID-19 on susceptibility to cancer [187]. In addition, according to the current evidence, SARS-CoV-2 may damage the prostate and worsen benign prostatic hyperplasia (BPH) and low urinary tracts (LUTS) via ACE2 signaling, androgen receptors (Ars)-related mechanisms, inflammation, and metabolic imbalance [188]. Because Ars has an important function in the pathophysiology of BPH and the infection of SARS-CoV-2 may be dependent on androgens, the progression of BPH and related symptoms is likely to be a complication of COVID-19 through the involvement of Ars and metabolic disorders. Therefore, future studies will be needed to investigate the possible role of COVID-19 in the progression of BPH–related LUTS and to examine prostate status in susceptible patients with available questionnaires (e.g., IPSS) and serum biomarkers (e.g., PSA).

Conclusion

The significant decline in male fertility and increasing incidence of cancer in the world represent a major concern for human health. Policymakers need to consider these relevant aspects, being supported by advanced health status monitoring systems, and undertake the necessary possible measures to protect health and well-being, especially in highly polluted areas, where male infertility and cancer incidence is higher.

We here underline the additive role of COVID-19 on sperm decline and its deleterious incidence on health in polluted areas and on cancer, which further increases worry when considering the effects on a younger population. Moreover, we aimed to highlight the role of spermatozoa as the first sentinels of the environmental health status thanks to their susceptibility to deleterious effects that may be triggered by environmental conditions, like pollution and pathogens infections, as in the case of SARS-CoV-2.

REFERENCES

1. Chen B, Kan H. Air pollution and population health: A global challenge. *Environ Health Prev Med* 2008;13(2):94–101.
2. Manisalidis I, Stavropoulou E, Stavropoulos A, Bezirtzoglou E. Environmental and health impacts of air pollution: A review. *Front Public Health* 2020:14.

3. EEA. Exceedance of air quality standards in urban areas. 2019. Available from: https://www.eea.europa.eu/data-and-maps/indicators/exceedance-of-air-quality-limit-3/assessment-5.

4. American Lung Association. American Lung Association State of the Air 2013 – Health Effects of Ozone and Particle Pollution. 2013. Available from: http://www.stateoftheair.org/2013/health-risks/.

5. Seaton A, Godden D, MacNee W, Donaldson K. Particulate air pollution and acute health effects. *The Lancet* 1995;345(8943):176–178.

6. Frampton MW, Stewart JC, Oberdorster G, et al. Inhalation of ultrafine particles alters blood leukocyte expression of adhesion molecules in humans. *Environ Health Perspect* 2006;114(1):51–58.

7. Wichmann D, Sperhake JP, Lütgehetmann M, et al. Autopsy findings and venous thromboembolism in patients with COVID-19: A prospective cohort study. *Ann Intern Med* 2020;173(4):268–277.

8. Ross MA. *Integrated science assessment for particulate matter.* US Environmental Protection Agency 2009. Washington, DC, pp. 61–161.

9. Russell AG, Brunekreef B. A focus on particulate matter and health. *Environ Sci Technol* 2009;43(13):4620–4625.

10. Vidale S, Bonanomi A, Guidotti M, et al. Air pollution positively correlates with daily stroke admission and in hospital mortality: A study in the urban area of Como, Italy. *Neurol Sci* 2010;31(2):179–182.

11. Hadei M, Naddafi K. Cardiovascular effects of airborne particulate matter: A review of rodent model studies. *Chemosphere* 2020;242:125204.

12. Tsai DH, Riediker M, Berchet A, et al. Effects of short- and long-term exposures to particulate matter on inflammatory marker levels in the general population. *Env Sci Pollut Res Int* 2019;26:19697–19704.

13. Araujo JA, Barajas B, Kleinman M, et al. Ambient particulate pollutants in the ultrafine range promote early atherosclerosis and systemic oxidative stress. *Circ Res* 2008;102:589–596.

14. Carlsen E, Giwercman A, Keiding N, et al. Evidence for decreasing quality of semen during past 50 years. *Br Med J* 1992;305:609–613.

15. Levine H, Jørgensen N, Martino-Andrade A, et al. Temporal trends in sperm count: A systematic review and meta-regression analysis. *Hum Reprod Update* 2017;23:646–659.

16. Levine H, Jørgensen N, Martino-Andrade A, et al. Temporal trends in sperm count: A systematic review and meta-regression analysis of samples collected globally in the 20th and 21st centuries. *Hum Reprod Update* 2022;1–20. https://doi.org/10.1093/humupd/dmac035.

17. Rehman S, Usman Z, Rehman S, et al. Endocrine disrupting chemicals and impact on male reproductive health. *Urol* 2018;7:490–503.

18. Lymperi S, Giwercman A. Endocrine disruptors and testicular function. *Metab Clin Exp* 2018;86:79–90.

19. Pironti C, Ricciardi M, Proto A, et al. Endocrine-disrupting compounds: An overview on their occurrence in the aquatic environment and human exposure. *Water* 2021;13:1347.

20. Deng, CF, Zhang M, et al. Association between air pollution and sperm quality: A systematic review and meta-analysis. *Environ Pollut* 2016;208:663–669.

21. Carré J, Gatimel N, Moreau J, et al. Does air pollution play a role in infertility? A systematic review. *Environ Health* 2017;16:82.

22. Wei Y, Cao XN, Tang XL, et al. Urban fine particulate matter (PM2.5) exposure destroys blood-testis barrier (BTB) integrity through excessive ros-mediated autophagy. *Toxicol Mech Methods* 2018;28:302–319.

23. Liu Y, Zhou Y, Ma J, et al. Inverse association between ambient sulfur dioxide exposure and semen quality in Wuhan, China. *Environ Sci Technol* 2017;51:12806–12814.

24. Gasparrini A. Modeling exposure-lag-response associations with distributed lag nonlinear models. *Stat Med* 2014;33:881–899.

25. Liu J, Ren L, Wei J, Zhang J, Zhu Y, Li X, Jing L, Duan J, Zhou X, Sun, Z. Fine particle matter disrupts the blood-testis barrier by activating TGF-B3/P38 MAPK pathway and decreasing testosterone secretion in rat. *Environ Toxicol* 2018;33:711–719.

26. Qiu L, Chen M, Wang X, Qin X, Chen S, Qian Y, Liu Z, Cao Q, Ying Z. Exposure to concentrated ambient PM2.5 compromises spermatogenesis in a mouse model: Role of suppression of hypothalamus-pituitary-gonads axis. *Toxicol Sci* 2018;162: 318–326.

27. Sun S, Zhao J, Cao W, et al. Identifying critical exposure windows for ambient air pollution and semen quality in Chinese men. *Environ Res* 2020;189:109894.

28. Bosco L, Notari T, Ruvolo G, Roccheri MC, Martino C, Chiappetta, R, Carone D, Lo Bosco G, Carrillo L, Raimondo S, et al. Sperm DNA fragmentation: An early and reliable marker of air pollution. *Environ Toxicol Pharmacol* 2018;58:243–249.

29. Vecoli C, Montano L, Andreassi MG. Environmental pollutants: Genetic damage and epigenetic changes in male germ cells. *Env Sci Pollut Res Int* 2016;23:23339–23348.

30. Eisenberg ML, Li S, Behr B, Pera RR, Cullen MR. Relationship between semen production and medical comorbidity. *Fertil Steril* 2015;103:66–71.

31. Choy JT, Eisenberg ML. Male infertility as a window to health. *Fertil Steril* 2018;110:810–814.

32. Glazer CH, Bonde JP, Eisenberg ML, Giwercman A, Hærvig KK, Rimborg S, Vassard D, Pinborg A, Schmidt L, Bräuner EV. Male infertility and risk of nonmalignant chronic diseases: A systematic review of the epidemiological evidence. *Semin Reprod Med* 2017;35:282–290.

33. Jensen TK, Jacobsen R, Christensen K, Nielsen NC, Bostofte E. Good semen quality and life expectancy: A cohort study of 43,277 men. *Am J Epidemiol* 2009;170:559–565.

34. Šrám RJ, Binková B, Rössner P, Rubeš J, Topinka J, Dejmek J. Adverse reproductive outcomes from exposure to environmental mutagens. *Mutat Res Fundam Mol Mech Mutagenesis* 1999;428:203–215.

35. Rubes J, Selevan SG, Evenson DP, Zudova D, Vozdova M, Zudova Z, Robbins WA, Perreault SD. Episodic air pollution is associated with increased DNA fragmentation in human sperm without other changes in semen quality. *Hum Reprod* 2005;20:2776–2783.

36. Jurewicz J, Radwan M, Sobala W, Polanska K, Radwan P, Jakubowski L, Ulánska A, Hanke W. The relationship between exposure to air pollution and sperm disomy. *Environ Mol Mutagen* 2015;56:50–59.

37. Lettieri G, D'Agostino G, Mele E, Cardito C, Esposito R, Cimmino A, Giarra A, Trifuoggi M, Raimondo S, Notari T, et al. Discovery of the involvement in DNA oxidative damage of human sperm nuclear basic proteins of healthy young men living in polluted areas. *Int J Mol Sci* 2020;21:4198.

38. Aitken RJ, Gibb Z, Baker MA, Drevet J, Gharagozloo P. Causes and consequences of oxidative stress in spermatozoa. *Reprod Fertil Dev* 2016;28:1–10.

39. Bergamo P, Volpe MG, Lorenzetti S, Mantovani A, Notari T, Cocca E, Cerullo S, Di Stasio M, Cerino P, Montano L. Human semen as an early, sensitive biomarker of highly polluted living environment in healthy men: A pilot biomonitoring study on trace elements in blood and semen and their relationship with sperm quality and RedOx status. *Reprod Toxicol* 2016;66:1–9.

40. Jurewicz J, Dziewirska E, Radwan M, Hanke W. Air pollution from natural and anthropic sources and male fertility. *Reprod Biol Endocrinol* 2018;16:109.
41. Montano L, Bergamo P, Andreassi MG, Vecoli C, Volpe MG, Lorenzetti S, Mantovani A, Notari T. The role of human semen for assessing environmental impact on human health in risk areas: Novels and early biomarkers of environmental pollution EcoFoodFertility Project. *Reprod Toxicol* 2017;72:44–45.
42. Vecoli C, Montano L, Borghini A, Notari T, Guglielmino A, Mercuri A, Turchi S, Andreassi MG. Effects of highly polluted environment on sperm telomere length: A pilot study. *Int J Mol Sci* 2017;18:1703.
43. Nowicka-Bauer K, Nixon, B. Molecular changes induced by oxidative stress that impair human sperm motility. *Antioxid* 2020 9;134.
44. Zhou P, Yang XL, Wang XG, et al. A pneumonia outbreak associated with a new coronavirus of probable bat origin. *Nature* 2020;579(7798):270–273.
45. Lin C-I, Tsai C-H, Sun Y-L, Hsieh W-Y, Lin Y-C, Chen C-Y, Lin C-S. Instillation of particulate matter 2.5 induced acute lung injury and attenuated the injury recovery in ACE2 knockout mice. *Int J Biol Sci* 2018;14:253–265.
46. Horan TS, Marre A, Hassold T, Lawson C, Hunt PA. Germline and reproductive tract effects intensify in male mice with successive generations of estrogenic exposure. *PLoS Genet* 2017;13:e1006885.
47. Lettieri G, Marra F, Moriello C, Prisco M, Notari T, Trifuoggi M, Giarra A, Bosco L, Montano L, Piscopo M. Molecular alterations in spermatozoa of a family case living in the land of fires. A first look at possible transgenerational effects of pollutants. *Int J Mol Sci* 2020;21:6710.
48. Post CM, Boule LA, Burke CG, O'Dell CT, Winans B, Lawrence BP. The ancestral environment shapes antiviral CD8+ T cell responses across. *Generations iScience* 2019;20:168–183.
49. Soubry A. POHaD: Why we should study future fathers. *Env Epigenet* 2018;4.
50. Xavier MJ, Roman SD, Aitken RJ, Nixon B. Transgenerational inheritance: How impacts to the epigenetic and genetic information of parents affect offspring health. *Hum Reprod Update* 2019;25:518–540.
51. Huangfu P, Atkinson R. Long-term exposure to NO2 and O3 and all-cause and respiratory mortality: A systematic review and meta-analysis. *Environ Int* 2020 November;144:105998. doi: 10.1016/j.envint.2020.105998. Epub 2020 October 5.
52. Chen J, Hoek G. Long-term exposure to PM and all-cause and cause-specific mortality: A systematic review and meta-analysis. *Environ Int* 2020 October;143:105974. doi: 10.1016/j.envint.2020.105974. Epub 2020 July 20.
53. Cheng I, et al. Traffic-related air pollution and lung cancer incidence: The California multiethnic cohort study. *Am J Respir Crit Care Med* 2022 October 15;206(8):1008–1018. doi: 10.1164/rccm.202107-1770OC.
54. Xue Y, Wang L, Zhang Y, Zhao Y, Liu Y. Air pollution: A culprit of lung cancer. *J Hazard Mater* 2022 July;15(434):128937. doi: 10.1016/j.jhazmat.2022.128937. Epub 2022 April 15.
55. Wong CM. Cancer mortality risks from long-term exposure to ambient fine particle. *Cancer Epidemiol Biomarkers Prev* 2016;25(5):839–845. https://doi.org/10.1158/1055-9965.EPI-15-0626
56. Pritchett N, Spangler EC, Gray GM, Livinski AA, Sampson JN, Dawsey SM, Jones RR. Exposure to outdoor particulate matter air pollution and risk of gastrointestinal cancers in adults: A systematic review and meta-analysis of epidemiologic evidence. *Environ Health Perspect* 2022 March;130(3):36001. doi: 10.1289/EHP9620. Epub 2022 March 2.

57. Mukherjee S, Dasgupta S, Mishra PK, Chaudhury K. Air pollution-induced epigenetic changes: Disease development and a possible link with hypersensitivity pneumonitis. *Environ Sci Pollut Res Int* 2021;28(40):55981–56002. doi: 10.1007/s11356-021-16056-x.

58. Chiusano ML. The modelling of COVID-19 pathways sheds light on mechanisms, opportunities and on controversial interpretations of medical treatments. 2022. https://arxiv.org/ftp/arxiv/papers/2003/2003.11614.

59. Montano L, Donato F, Bianco PM, et al Air pollution and COVID-19: A possible dangerous synergy for male fertility. *Int J Environ Res Public Health* 2021;18:6846. https://doi.org/10.3390/ijerph18136846.

60. Muhanna D, Arnipalli SR, Kumar SB, et al. Osmotic adaptation by Na^+-dependent transporters and ACE2: Correlation with hemostatic crisis in COVID-19. *Biomedicines* 2020;8:460.

61. Costanzo L, Grasso SA, Palumbo FP, Ardita G, Di Pino L, Antignani PL, Aluigi L, Arosio E, Failla G. 2020. Pneumopatia da COVID-19: il punto di vista del Medico Vascolare. http://www.sidv.net/file_doc/Pneumopatia%20da%20COVID%20for%20SIDV%20finale.pdf.

62. Burstein SA. Cytokines, platelet production and hemostasis. *Platelets* 1997;8(2–3): 93–104.

63. Esmon CT, Fukudome K, Mather T, et al. Inflammation, sepsis, and coagulation. *Haematologica* 1999;84(3):254–259.

64. Esmon CT. The interactions between inflammation and coagulation. *Br J Haematol* 2005 November;131(4):417–430. doi: 10.1111/j.1365-2141.2005.05753.x.

65. McKay DG, Margaretten W. Disseminated intravascular coagulation in virus diseases. *Arch Intern Med* 1967;120(2):129–152.

66. Li H, Liu S, Yu XH, et al. Coronavirus disease 2019 (COVID-19): Current status and future perspectives. *Int J Antimicrob Agents* 2020;55:105951.

67. Varga Z, Flammer AJ, Steiger P, et al. Endothelial cell infection and endotheliitis in COVID-19. *Lancet* 2020;395:1417–1418.

68. Short KR, Veeris R, Leijten LM, et al. Proinflammatory cytokine responses in extrarespiratory tissues during severe influenza. *J Infect Dis* 2017;216:829–833.

69. Ludlow M, Kortekaas J, Herden C, et al. Neurotropic virus infections as the cause of immediate and delayed neuropathology. *Acta Neuropathol* 2016;131:159–184.

70. Libbey JE, Kennett NJ, Wilcox KS, et al. Interleukin-6, produced by resident cells of the central nervous system and infiltrating cells, contributes to the development of seizures following viral infection. *J Virol* 2011;85:6913–6922.

71. Probert L. TNF and its receptors in the CNS: The essential, the desirable and the deleterious effects. *Neuroscience* 2015;302:2–22.

72. Caso F, Costa L, Ruscitti P, et al. Could sars-coronavirus-2 trigger autoimmune and/or autoinflammatory mechanisms in genetically predisposed subjects? *Autoimmun Rev* 2020;19:102524.

73. Masters SL, Simon A, Aksentijevich I, et al. Horror autoinflammaticus: The molecular pathophysiology of autoinflammatory disease. *Annu Rev Immunol* 2009;27: 621–668.

74. Tanaka T, Narazaki M, Kishimoto T. IL-6 in Inflammation, Immunity, and Disease. *Cold Spring Harb Perspect Biol* 2014;6:a016295.

75. El-Maadawy EA, Talaat RM, Ahmed MM, et al. Interleukin-6 promotor gene polymorphisms and susceptibility to chronic hepatitis B virus in Egyptians. *Hum Immunol* 2019;80:208–214.

76. Saper VE, Chen G, Deutsch GH, et al. Emergent high fatality lung disease in systemic juvenile arthritis. *Ann Rheum Dis* 2019;78:1722–1731.

77. Schulert GS, Yasin S, Carey B, et al. Systemic juvenile idiopathic arthritis-associated lung disease: Characterization and risk factors. *Arthritis Rheumatol* 2019;71:1943–1954.
78. Mehta P, McAuley DF, Brown M, et al. COVID-19: Consider cytokine storm syndromes and immunosuppression. *Lancet* 2020;395:1033–1034.
79. Ramos-Casals M, Brito-Zerón P, López-Guillermo A, et al. Adult haemophagocytic syndrome. *Lancet* 2014;383:1503–1516.
80. Frontera A, Martin C, Vlachos K, et al. Regional air pollution persistence links to COVID-19 infection zoning. *J Infect* 2020;81:318–356.
81. Bontempi E. Commercial exchanges instead of air pollution as possible origin of COVID-19 initial diffusion phase in Italy: More efforts are necessary to address interdisciplinary research. *Environ Res* 2020;188:109775.
82. Lin K, Yee-Tak Fong D, Zhu B, et al. Environmental factors on the SARS epidemic: Air temperature, passage of time and multiplicative effect of hospital infection. *Epidemiol Infect* 2006;134:223–230.
83. Qin N, Liang P, Wu C, et al. Longitudinal survey of microbiome associated with particulate matter in a megacity. *Genome Biol* 2020;21:55.
84. Tung NT, Cheng P-C. Chi K, et al. Particulate matter and SARS-CoV-2: A possible model of COVID-19 transmission. *Sci Total Env* 2021;750:141532.
85. Ram K, Thakur RC, Singh DK, Et al. Why airborne transmission hasn't been conclusive in case of COVID-19? An atmospheric science perspective. *Sci Total Environ* 2021;773:145525.
86. Cui Y, Zhang ZF, Froines J, et al. Air pollution and case fatality of SARS in the People's Republic of China: An ecologic study. *Env Health* 2003;2:15.
87. Yao Y, Pan J, Liu Z, et al. Temporal association between particulate matter pollution and case fatality rate of COVID-19 in Wuhan. *Environ Res* 2020;189:109941.
88. Sarkodie SA, Owusu PA. Global effect of city-to-city air pollution, health conditions, climatic & socio-economic factors on COVID-19 pandemic. *Sci Total Env* 2021; 778:146394.
89. Wu X, Nethery RC, Sabath MB, et al. Air pollution and COVID-19 mortality in the United States: Strengths and limitations of an ecological regression analysis. *Sci Adv* 2020;6(45): eabd4049.
90. Ali N, Islam F. The effects of air pollution on COVID-19 infection and mortality – A review on recent evidence. *Front Public Health* 2020;8:580057.
91. Comunian S, Dongo D, Milani C, et al. Air pollution and COVID-19: The role of particulate matter in the spread and increase of COVID-19's morbidity and mortality. *Int J Environ Res Public Health* 2020;17:4487.
92. Mukherjee, BS, Siddiqi H, et al. Present cum future of SARS-CoV-2 virus and its associated control of virus-laden air pollutants leading to potential environmental threat – A global review. *J Environ Chem Eng* 2021;9:104973.
93. Martelletti L, Martelletti P. Air pollution and the novel COVID-19 disease: A putative disease risk factor. *SN Compr Clin Med* 2020;2:383–387.
94. Fattorini D, Regoli F. Role of the chronic air pollution levels in the COVID-19 outbreak risk in italy. *Environ Pollut* 2020;264:114e732.
95. Ogen Y. Assessing nitrogen dioxide (NO2) levels as a contributing factor to coronavirus (COVID-19) fatality. *Sci Total Environ* 2020;726:138605.
96. Pozzer, A, Dominici F, Haines A, et al. Regional and global contributions of air pollution to risk of death from COVID-19. *Cardiovasc Res* 2020;116:2247–2253.
97. Brini L, Hiri S, Ijaz M, et al.. Temporal and climate characteristics of respiratory syncytial virus bronchiolitis in neonates and children in Sousse, Tunisia, during a 13-year surveillance. *Env Sci Pollut Res* 2020;27:23379–23389.

98. Zhou N, Cui Z, Yang S, et al. Air pollution and decreased semen quality: A comparative study of Chongqing urban and rural areas. *Environ Pollut* 2014;187:145–152.
99. Nordkap L, Joensen UN, Blomberg JM, et al. Regional differences and temporal trends in male reproductive health disorders: Semen quality may be a sensitive marker of environmental exposures. *Mol Cell Endocrinol* 2012;355:221–230.
100. Le Moal J, Rolland M, Goria S, Royère D. Semen quality trends in French regions are consistent with a global change in environmental exposure. *Reproduction* 2014;147:567–574.
101. Casas M, Chevrier C, Hond ED, et al. Exposure to brominated flame retardants, perfluorinated compounds, phthalates and phenols in European birth cohorts: ENRIECO evaluation, first human biomonitoring results, and recommendations. *Int J Hyg Environ Health* 2013;216:230–242.
102. Bergman A, Heindel JJ, Kasten T, Kidd KA, Jobling S, Neira M, Zoeller RT, Becher G, Bjerregaard P, Bornman R, et al. The impact of endocrine disruption: A consensus statement on the state of the science. *Environ Health Perspect* 2013;121:A104–A106.
103. Sajadi MM, Habibzadeh P, Vintzileos A, Shokouhi S, Miralles-Wilhelm F, Amoroso A. Temperature, humidity, and latitude analysis to estimate potential spread and seasonality of coronavirus disease 2019 (COVID-19). *JAMA Netw Open* 2020;3(6):e2011834–e2011834.
104. Lettieri G, Mollo V, Ambrosino A, Caccavale F, Troisi J, Febbraio F, Piscopo M. Molecular effects of copper on the reproductive system of *mytilus galloprovincialis*. *Mol Reprod Dev* 2019;86:1357–1368.
105. Piscopo M, Notariale R, Rabbito D, Ausió J, Olanrewaju OS, Guerriero G. *Mytilus galloprovincialis* (Lamarck, 1819) spermatozoa: Hsp70 expression and protamine-like protein property studies. *Env Sci Pollut Res Int* 2018;25:12957–12966.
106. Piscopo M, Trifuoggi M, Notariale R, Labar S, Troisi J, Giarra A, Rabbito D, Puoti R, de Benedictis D, Brundo MV, et al. Protamine-like proteins' analysis as an emerging biotechnique for cadmium impact assessment on male mollusk *mytilus galloprovincialis* (Lamarck 1819). *Acta Biochim Pol* 2018;65:259–267.
107. De Guglielmo V, Puoti R, Notariale R, Maresca V, Ausió J, Troisi J, Verrillo M, Basile A, Febbraio F, Piscopo M. Alterations in the properties of sperm protamine-like II protein after exposure of *mytilus galloprovincialis* (Lamarck 1819) to sub-toxic doses of cadmium. *Ecotoxicol Environ Saf* 2019;169:600–606.
108. Montano L, Donato F, Bianco PM, Lettieri G, Guglielmino A, Motta O, Bonapace IM, Piscopo M. Semen quality as a potential susceptibility indicator to SARS-CoV-2 insults in polluted areas. *Environ Sci Pollut Res* 2021;28(28): 37031–37040.
109. Montano L. Reproductive biomarkers as early indicators for assessing environmental health risk. In Marfe, G, and Di Stefano C. *Toxic Waste Management and Health Risk*, BenthamScience Publishers eBook eISBN 978-981-14-5474-5, 2020. doi: 10.2174/9789811454745120010.1. https://www.eurekaselect.com/185279/chapter112.
110. Reis AB, Araújo FC, Pereira VM, et al. Angiotensin (1–7) and its receptor mas are expressed in the human testis: Implications for male infertility. *J Mol Histol* 2010;41:75–80.
111. Borro M, Di Girolamo P, Gentile G. Evidence-based considerations exploring relations between SARS-CoV-2 pandemic and air pollution: Involvement of PM2.5-mediated up-regulation of the viral receptor ACE-2. *Int J Environ Res Public Health* 2020;17:5573.
112. Frontera A, Cianfanelli L, Vlachos K, et al. Air pollution links to higher mortality in COVID-19 patients: The "double-hit" hypothesis. *J Infect* 2020;81:255–259.

113. Dejucq N, Jégou B. Viruses in the mammalian male genital tract and their effects on the reproductive system. *Microbiol Mol Biol Rev* 2001;65:208–231.

114. Shen Q, Xiao X, Aierken A, et al. The ACE2 expression in Sertoli cells and germ cells may cause male reproductive disorder after SARS-CoV-2 infection. *J Cell Mol Med* 2020;24(16):9472–9477.

115. Glencross DA, Ho T-R, Camiña N, Hawrylowicz CM, Pfeffer PE. Air pollution and its effects on the immune system. *Free Radic Biol Med* 2020;151:56–68.

116. Breton CV, Song AY, Xiao J, Kim S-J, Mehta HH, Wan J, Yen K, Sioutas C, Lurmann F, Xue S, et al. Effects of air pollution on mitochondrial function, mitochondrial DNA methylation, and mitochondrial peptide expression. *Mitochondrion* 2019;46:22–29.

117. Wu S, McGoogan JF. Characteristics of and important lessons from the coronavirus disease 2019 (COVID-19) outbreak in China: Summary of a report of 72,314 cases from the Chinese center for disease control and prevention. *JAMA* 2020;April 7;323(13):1239–1242. doi: 10.1001/jama.2020.2648.

118. Sica A, Colombo MP, Trama A, et al. Immunometabolic status of COVID-19 cancer patients *Physiol Rev* 2020 October 1;100(4):1839–1850. doi: 10.1152/physrev.00018.2020.

119. Dai M, Liu D, Liu M, et al. Patients with cancer appear more vulnerable to SARS-CoV-2: A multicenter study during the COVID-19 outbreak. *Cancer Discov* 2020;10:783–791.

120. Sacks D, Baxter B, Campbell BCV, et al. Multisociety consensus quality improvement revised consensus statement for endovascular therapy of acute ischemic stroke. *Int J Stroke* 2018 August;13(6):612–632. doi: 10.1177/1747493018778713.

121. Rolla R, Chiara Puricelli C, Alessandra BA, et al. Platelets: "Multiple choice" effectors in the immune response and their implication in COVID-19 thromboinflammatory process. *Int J Lab Hematol* 2021 October;43(5):895–906.

122. Lunski MJ, Burton J, Tawagi K, et al. Multivariate mortality analyses in COVID-19: Comparing patients with cancer and patients without cancer in Louisiana. *Cancer* 2021;127:266.

123. Bertuzzi AF, Ciccarelli M, Marrari A, et al. Impact of active cancer on COVID-19 survival: A matched-analysis on 557 consecutive patients at an Academic Hospital in Lombardy, *Italy Br J Cancer* 2021;125:358.

124. Fu C, Stoeckle JH, Masri L, et al. COVID-19 outcomes in hospitalized patients with active cancer: Experiences from a major New York City health care system. *Cancer* 2021;127:3466.

125. Docherty AB, Harrison EM, Green CA, et al. Features of 20 133 UK patients in hospital with COVID-19 using the ISARIC WHO clinical characterisation protocol: Prospective observational cohort study. *BMJ* 2020;369:m1985.

126. Brar G, Pinheiro LC, Shusterman M, et al. COVID-19 severity and outcomes in patients with cancer: A matched cohort study. *J Clin Oncol* 2020;38:3914.

127. Sengar M, Chinnaswamy G, Ranganathan P, et al. Outcomes of COVID-19 and risk factors in patients with cancer. *Nat Cancer* 2022;3:547.

128. OnCovid Study Group, Pinato DJ, Patel M, et al. Time-dependent COVID-19 mortality in patients with cancer: An updated analysis of the OnCovid registry. *JAMA Oncol* 2022;8:114.

129. Williamson EJ, Walker AJ, Bhaskaran K, et al. Factors associated with COVID-19-related death using OpenSAFELY. *Nature* 2020;584:430.

130. Mehta V, Goel S, Kabarriti R, et al. Case fatality rate of cancer patients with COVID-19 in a New York hospital system. *Cancer Discov* 2020;10:93.

131. Cai Y, Hao Z, Gao Y, et al. Coronavirus disease 2019 in the perioperative period of lung resection: A brief report from a single thoracic surgery department in Wuhan, People's Republic of China. *J Thorac Oncol* 2020;15:1065.
132. Luo J, Rizvi H, Preeshagul IR, et al. COVID-19 in patients with lung cancer. *Ann Oncol* 2020;31:1386.
133. Horn L, Whisenant JG, Torri V, et al. Thoracic cancers international COVID-19 collaboration (TERAVOLT): Impact of type of cancer therapy and COVID therapy on survival. *J Clin Oncol* 2020;LBA111–LBA111.
134. Johnston EE, Martinez I, Davis ES, et al. SARS-CoV-2 in childhood cancer in 2020: A disease of disparities. *J Clin Oncol* 2021;39:3778.
135. Whisenant JG, Baena J, Cortellini A, et al. A definitive prognostication system for patients with thoracic malignancies diagnosed with coronavirus disease 2019: An update from the TERAVOLT registry. *J Thorac Oncol* 2022;17:661.
136. Várnai C, Palles C, Arnold R, et al. Mortality among adults with cancer undergoing chemotherapy or immunotherapy and infected with COVID-19. *JAMA Netw Open* 2022;5:e220130.
137. Mileham KF, Bruinooge SS, Aggarwal C, et al. Changes over time in COVID-19 severity and mortality in patients undergoing cancer treatment in the United States: Initial report from the ASCO registry. *JCO Oncol Pract* 2022;18:e426.
138. Khoury E, Nevitt S, Madsen WR, et al. Differences in outcomes and factors associated with mortality among patients with SARS-CoV-2 infection and cancer compared with those without cancer: A systematic review and meta-analysis. *JAMA Netw Open* 2022;5:e2210880.
139. Han X, Hu X, Zhao J, et al. Identification of deaths caused by cancer and COVID-19 in the US during March to December 2020. *JAMA Oncol* 2022;8:1696.
140. Gong IY, Vijenthira A, Powis M, et al. Association of COVID-19 vaccination with breakthrough infections and complications in patients with cancer. *JAMA Oncol* 2022 December 29. doi: 10.1001/jamaoncol.2022.6815.
141. Falanga A, Marchetti M, Vignoli A. Coagulation and cancer: Biological and clinical aspects. *J Thromb Haemost* 2013;Februry;11(2):223–233. doi: 10.1111/jth.12075.
142. Rostami M, Hassan Mansouritorghabeh H. D-dimer level in COVID-19 infection: A systematic review. *Expert Rev Hematol* 2020 November;13(11):1265–1275. doi: 10.1080/17474086.2020.1831383.12.
143. Ripon AR, Bhowmik DR, Amin MT, et al. Role of arachidonic cascade in COVID-19 infection: A review. *Prostaglandins Other Lipid Mediat* 2021 January;154:106539. doi: 10.1016/j.prostaglandins.2021.106539.
144. Snider JM, You JK,, Wang X, et al. Group IIA secreted phospholipase A2 is associated with the pathobiology leading to COVID-19 mortality. *J Clin Invest* 2021 October 1;131(19):e149236. doi: 10.1172/JCI149236.
145. Brogna C, Barbara Brogna B, Domenico Rocco Bisaccia DR, et al. Could SARS-CoV-2 have bacteriophage behavior or induce the activity of other bacteriophages? *Vaccines* 2022 April 29;10(5):708. doi: 10.3390/vaccines10050708.
146. Plaza-Díaz J, Ana I Álvarez-Mercado AI, Carmen M Ruiz-Marín CM, et al. Association of breast and gut microbiota dysbiosis and the risk of breast cancer: A case-control clinical study. *BMC Cancer* 2019 May 24;19(1):495. doi: 10.1186/s12885-019-5660-y.
147. Mingyang Song M, Andrew T Chan AT, Jun SJ. Influence of the gut microbiome, diet, and environment on risk of colorectal cancer. *Gastroenterology* 2020 January;158(2):322–340. doi: 10.1053/j.gastro.2019.06.048. Epub 2019 October 3.

148. Rugge M ZMaGS. SARS-CoV-2 infection in the Italian Veneto region: Adverse outcomes in patients with cancer. *Nature Cancer* 2020;1: 784–8:58.

149. Sanchez-Pina JM, Rodriguez Rodriguez M, Castro Quismondo N, et al. Clinical course and risk factors for mortality from COVID-19 in patients with haematological malignancies. *Eur J Haematol* 2020;105:597–607.

150. Giannakoulis VG, Papoutsi E, Siempos II. Effect of cancer on clinical outcomes of patients with COVID-19: A meta-analysis of patient data. *JCO Glob Oncol* 2020;6:799.

151. Tian J, Yuan X, Xiao J, et al. Clinical characteristics and risk factors associated with COVID-19 disease severity in patients with cancer in Wuhan, China: A multicentre, retrospective, cohort study. *Lancet Oncol* 2020;21:893.

152. Passamonti F, Cattaneo C, Arcaini L, et al. Clinical characteristics and risk factors associated with COVID-19 severity in patients with haematological malignancies in Italy: A retrospective, multicentre, cohort study. *Lancet Haematol* 2020;7:e737.

153. Kuderer NM, Choueiri TK, Shah DP, et al. Clinical impact of COVID-19 on patients with cancer (CCC19): A cohort study. *Lancet* 2020;395:1907.

154. Albiges L, Foulon S, Bayle A, et al. Determinants of the outcomes of patients with cancer infected with SARS-CoV-2: Results from the Gustave Roussy cohort. *Nat Cancer* 2020;1:965.

155. Pinato DJ, Zambelli A, Aguilar-Company J, et al. Clinical portrait of the SARS-CoV-2 epidemic in European cancer patients. *Cancer Discov* 2020 July 31;10(10):1465–1474. doi: 10.1158/2159-8290.CD-20-0773.

156. Jee J, Foote MB, Lumish M, et al. Chemotherapy and COVID-19 outcomes in patients with cancer. *J Clin Oncol* 2020;38:3538.

157. Fox TA, Troy-Barnes E, Kirkwood AA, et al. Clinical outcomes and risk factors for severe COVID-19 in patients with haematological disorders receiving chemo- or immunotherapy. *Br J Haematol* 2020;191:194.

158. Fillmore NR, La J, Szalat RE, et al. Prevalence and outcome of COVID-19 infection in cancer patients: A national Veterans Affairs study. *J Natl Cancer Inst* 2021;113:691.

159. Garassino MC, Whisenant JG, Huang LC, et al. COVID-19 in patients with thoracic malignancies (TERAVOLT): First results of an international, registry-based, cohort study. *Lancet Oncol* 2020;21(7):914–922.

160. Yekedüz E, Utkan G, Ürün Y. A systematic review and meta-analysis: The effect of active cancer treatment on severity of COVID-19. *Eur J Cancer* 2020;141:92.

161. Robilotti EV, Babady NE, Mead PA, et al. Determinants of COVID-19 disease severity in patients with cancer. *Nat Med* 2020;26:1218.

162. Pinato DJ, Tabernero J, Bower M, et al. Prevalence and impact of COVID-19 sequelae on treatment and survival of patients with cancer who recovered from SARS-CoV-2 infection: Evidence from the OnCovid retrospective, multicentre registry study. *Lancet Oncol* 2021;22:1669.

163. Lee LY, Cazier JB, Angelis V, et al. COVID-19 mortality in patients with cancer on chemotherapy or other anticancer treatments: A prospective cohort study. *Lancet* 2020;395:1919.

164. Wang Q, Berger NA, Xu R. Analyses of risk, racial disparity, and outcomes among US Patients with cancer and COVID-19 infection. *JAMA Oncol* 2021;7:220.

165. Saini KS, Tagliamento M, Lambertini M, et al. Mortality in patients with cancer and coronavirus disease 2019: A systematic review and pooled analysis of 52 studies. *Eur J Cancer* 2020;139:43.

166. Cook G, John Ashcroft A, Pratt G, et al. Real-world assessment of the clinical impact of symptomatic infection with severe acute respiratory syndrome coronavirus (COVID-19 disease) in patients with multiple myeloma receiving systemic anti-cancer therapy. *Br J Haematol* 2020;190:e83.
167. Singh AK, Gillies CL, Singh R, et al. Prevalence of co-morbidities and their association with mortality in patients with COVID-19: A systematic review and meta-analysis. *Diabetes Obes Metab* 2020;22(1915).
168. Van Doesum J, Chinea A, Pagliaro M, et al. Clinical characteristics and outcome of SARS-CoV-2-infected patients with haematological diseases: A retrospective case study in four hospitals in Italy, Spain and the Netherlands. *Leukemia* 2020;34:2536.
169. Grasselli G, Greco M, Zanella A, et al. Risk factors associated with mortality among patients with COVID-19 in intensive care units in Lombardy, Italy. *JAMA Intern Med* 2020;180:1345.
170. Lee LYW, Cazier JB, Starkey T, et al. COVID-19 prevalence and mortality in patients with cancer and the effect of primary tumour subtype and patient demographics: A prospective cohort study. *Lancet Oncol* 2020;21:1309.
171. Zhou Y, Yang Q, Chi J, et al. Comorbidities and the risk of severe or fatal outcomes associated with coronavirus disease 2019: A systematic review and meta-analysis. *Int J Infect Dis* 2020;99:47.
172. Zhang H, Han H, He T, et al. Clinical characteristics and outcomes of COVID-19-infected cancer patients: A systematic review and meta-analysis. *J Natl Cancer Inst* 2021;113:371.
173. Barek MA, Aziz MA, Islam MS. Impact of age, sex, comorbidities and clinical symptoms on the severity of COVID-19 cases: A meta-analysis with 55 studies and 10014 cases. *Heliyon* 2020;6:e05684.
174. Jiang C, Yabroff KR, Deng L, et al. Prevalence of underlying medical conditions associated with severe COVID-19 illness in adult cancer survivors in the United States. *J Natl Cancer Inst* 2022;114:156.
175. Parker RS, Le J, Doan A, et al. COVID-19 outcomes in children, adolescents and young adults with cancer. *Int J Cancer* 2022;151:1913.
176. Mangone L, Gioia F, Mancuso P, et al. Cumulative COVID-19 incidence, mortality and prognosis in cancer survivors: A population-based study in Reggio Emilia, Northern Italy. *Int J Cancer* 2021 April 16;149(4):820–826. doi: 10.1002/ijc.33601.
177. Gupta S, Sutradhar R, Alexander S, Science M. Risk of COVID-19 infections and of severe complications among survivors of childhood, adolescent, and young adult cancer: A population-based study in Ontario, Canada. *J Clin Oncol* 2022 April 20;40(12):1281–1290. doi: 10.1200/JCO.21.02592. Epub 2022 Februry 28.
178. Kadan-Lottick NS, Vanderwerker LC, Block SD, et al. Psychiatric disorders and mental health service use in patients with advanced cancer. *Cancer* 2005 December 15;104(12):2872–2881. doi: 10.1002/cncr.21532.
179. Zeber JE, Copeland LA, Hosek BJ, et al. Cancer rates, medical comorbidities, and treatment modalities in the oldest patients, *Crit Rev Oncol Hematol* 2008;67(3):237–242.
180. Sica A, Colombo MP, Trama A, et al. Immunometaolic status of COVID-19 cancer patients. *Physiol Rev* 2020;100:1839–1850 July 28, Downloaded from journals. physiology.org/journal/physrev (151.077.150.225) on January 22, 2023.
181. Rogado J, Pangua C, Serrano-Montero G, et al. COVID-19 and lung cancer: A greater fatality rate? *Lung Cancer* 2020;146:19–22.

182. The OpenSAFELY Collaborative, Williamson E, Walker AJ, Bhaskaran K, et al. OpenSAFELY: Factors associated with COVID-19–related hospital death in the linked electronic health records of 17 million adult NHS patients (Preprint). medRxiv 2020.05.06.20092999, 2020. doi:10.1101/2020.05.06.20092999.
183. Khawaja AP, Warwick AN, Hysi PG, et al. Associations with COVID-19 hospitalisation amongst 406,793 adults: The UK Biobank prospective cohort study. MedRxiv 2020. https://doi.org/10.1101/2020.05.06.20092957.
184. Zhang L, Zhu F, Xie L, et al. Clinical characteristics of COVID-19-infected cancer patients: A retrospective case study in three hospitals within Wuhan, China. *Ann Oncol* 2020;31:894–901.
185. Gourd E. New evidence that air pollution contributes substantially to lung cancer. *Lancet Oncol* 2022 October;23(10):e448. doi: 10.1016/S1470-2045(22)00569-1.
186. Anup S Pathania AS, Prathipati P, Abdul RA COVID-19 and cancer comorbidity: Therapeutic opportunities and challenges. *Theranostics* 2021 January 1;11(2):731–753. https://doi.org/10.7150/thno.51471.eCollection 2021.
187. Saini G, Aneja R. Cancer as a prospective sequela of long COVID-19. *Bioessays* 2021 January;43(6):e2000331. doi: 10.1002/bies.202000331.
188. Haghpanah A, Masjedi F, Salehipour M, et al. Is COVID-19 a risk factor for progression of benign prostatic hyperplasia and exacerbation of its related symptoms? A systematic review. *Prostate Cancer Prostatic Dis* 2022 March;25(1):27–38. doi: 10.1038/s41391-021-00388-3.

Index

Pages in *italics* refer to figures and pages in **bold** refer to tables.

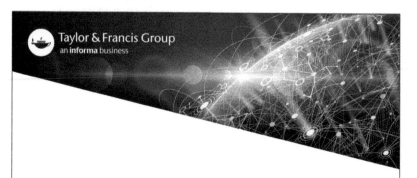

Taylor & Francis eBooks

www.taylorfrancis.com

A single destination for eBooks from Taylor & Francis with increased functionality and an improved user experience to meet the needs of our customers.

90,000+ eBooks of award-winning academic content in Humanities, Social Science, Science, Technology, Engineering, and Medical written by a global network of editors and authors.

TAYLOR & FRANCIS EBOOKS OFFERS:

A streamlined experience for our library customers

A single point of discovery for all of our eBook content

Improved search and discovery of content at both book and chapter level

REQUEST A FREE TRIAL
support@taylorfrancis.com

 Routledge
Taylor & Francis Group

 CRC Press
Taylor & Francis Group

Milton Keynes UK
Ingram Content Group UK Ltd.
UKHW022041141024
449569UK00014B/677

9 781032 423838